The Kitchen Table Book:

1,427 Kitchen Cures and Pantry Potions for Just About Every Health and Household Problem

Publisher's Note

Heal me, O Lord, and I will be healed; save me and I will be saved,
for You are my praise.

Jeremiah 17:14

FC&A Medical Publishing®
103 Clover Green
Peachtree City, GA 30269

Produced by the staff of FC&A

ISBN 978-1-932470-92-5

Table of Contents

Açai
Rescue your health with the latest 'superfood' 1

Apples
Get to the core of cancer protection 4
Snack on the 'super fruit' that's good for your heart 5
Bone up on your diet's missing link 6
Pump up the fiber for a great gut 7
An apple a day keeps memory safe 8
Give your lungs a powerful boost 9

Aspirin
Save yourself from a hidden stroke threat 11
Beat cancer at the backyard grill 12
Aspirin a day keeps 3 health threats away 13
Uncover the truth about buffered aspirin 16

Baking soda
Clear your sinuses without drugs 17
Take the ouch out of bites and stings .18
Scrub away food poisoning peril 19
Cheap solution for head-to-toe grooming 20
Kitchen staple cleans house top to bottom 21

Bananas
Lower your blood pressure without pills 23
Shut off your brain for better sleep 24
Calm your irritable gut 25
Give your bones royal protection 26

Beans
Fifty-cent food tames cancer 28
Simple way to sack type 2 diabetes 30
Half a cup does your heart good 31

Beta carotene
Heal your heart with a food rainbow 33
Pumpkins put the squeeze on cancer .35
Take a bite out of Alzheimer's 37
Get fitter without moving a muscle 37
Potatoes protect peepers from blindness 39
Breathe easier with beta carotene 41

Black tea

Enjoy a bonanza for your bones 42
More tea means less cancer 43
5 ways tea fights heart disease 44
Drink your stress away 45
Easy way to combat colds and flu 47
Nip cavities in the bud 48

Blood orange

Go red for great health 49

Breakfast cereal

Eat breakfast to blast belly fat 52
A bowl a day keeps diabetes at bay 54
$4 secret to preventing heart disease 55
Get regular with the right cereal 57

Capsaicin

Cool chronic pain with hot peppers 59
Douse the burn of indigestion 61
Dash of cayenne crushes cancer 63
Spicy seasoning melts away pounds 64
Turn up the heat to beat diabetes 65

Cherries

Ease arthritis pain with an everyday fruit 66
Guard your heart with inflammation fighters 67
Little fruit packs a wallop against cancer 68

Chocolate

Tasty treat heads off heart disease 69
Dark chocolate drops high blood pressure 71
Sweet solution to staying sharp 72
Drink cocoa to look years younger 74
Chocolate busts deadly blood clots 74

Cinnamon

Spice up your blood sugar control 77
Heart health: a new reason to season .78
Scent-sational safety tip 79

Citrus

Go orange to save your pearly whites 80
'C' how citrus battles diabetes 82
Cancer cure is no pulp fiction 84
Juice up your joint and bone protection 85
7 terrific tips for nontoxic cleaning 88

Coffee

Filter out two kinds of cancer 88
Ward off diabetes with a daily java jolt 89
Coffee breaks won't break your heart 92
Coffee perk: less risk of Alzheimer's 93

Cornstarch

Bedtime snack balances blood sugar 95
Soothe skin with silky solution 97

Cranberries

Wash away bacteria for all-over health 99
Little red berry offers triple defense .101
Berry breakthrough in cancer battle .102

Cruciferous vegetables

Tender sprouts safeguard bladder 104
Beat the odds against breast cancer .105
Brassicas K.O. colon cancer 107
Common cabbage keeps arthritis at bay 108
Boost your immune system with broccoli 110
Pile on the veggies for prostate health 111

Curry powder

Golden spice keeps your brain sharp 112
Savor a spicy cancer fighter 113
Follow the yellow brick road to diabetes defense 114
Protect your heart with curry power .117

Dairy

Delicious way to dodge diabetes 117
Burn fat faster with a creamy treat 119
Uncover the truth about milk and bones 121
Dairy: the answer to colon cancer 122

Eggs

Fit eggs into a heart-smart diet 123
Breakfast trick melts pounds and inches 126

Fish

Help yourself to heart-healthy fish 127
Powerful weapon protects against stroke 129
Fight diabetes with a fishy food plan 130
Easy way to boost your brainpower .131
Brighten your mood with seafood 133
Keep an eye on fish for better vision 134
Surround your joints with gentle relief 135

Fish *(continued)*
    Soothe inflammatory bowel disease 137
    Catch a fish and catch your breath 138
    Fortify your body against disease 139

Flaxseed
    Super seed saves your heart 141
    Easy way to protect your prostate 143
    2 terrific ways to help your head 144

Garlic
    Amazing herb helps your heart 147
    Garlic slashes cancer risk 149
    Bulb boosts immune system 150
    Dodge diabetes with garlic 151
    Surprising way to treat UTIs 151

Ginger
    Take a detour from queasy street 153
    Fight dangerous inflammation with ginger 154

Goji berry
    Ancient Chinese superfruit protects your vision 157
    Stay young with goji power 158

Green tea
    Nip cavities in the bud 160
    Drink up to keep blood sugar down .161
    Sip a summer skin saver 162
    Easy way to keep your memory sharp 164
    Go green to prevent inflammation 166
    Latest scoop on tea and prostate cancer 166

Honey
    Discover the healing wonder of honey 169
    Beat insomnia with this sleeper hit .171
    Heal your body inside and out 171
    Guard your heart with a simple switch 173
    Head off pollen problems 174

Inulin
    3 ways inulin protects your colon 176
    Simple sugar fits diabetes diet 177

Leafy greens
    4 powerful ways to fend off heart disease 179
    Keep your memory sharp as a tack 180
    2 ways greens keep your body young 183

5-a-day plan beats cancer 183
Enjoy a triple defense against cancer 186
Go green for a healthy prostate 186

Lutein & zeaxanthin
Fight vision loss and win 187
Wise way to counteract cataracts 188
Foil a future heart attack 189

Magnesium
Balance blood sugar with a marvelous mineral 190
Pathway to lower blood pressure and a healthy heart 191
Cancel out colon cancer 192
Mag-nificent way to better health 194

Mangosteen
Unusual fruit promises top defense 195
Superfruit keeps you super fresh 197

Nuts
Say 'nuts' to a heart attack 198
Nutty way to fight diabetes 201
The real truth about nuts and weight 202

Oatmeal
Basic breakfast guards your heart 203
Slimming oats help you watch your waistline 205
Balance blood sugar with a breakfast basic 206
Enjoy clearer, younger-looking skin 208
New hope for celiac disease 209

Olive oil
Change your oil for a healthier heart 211
Oil your joints for soothing relief 212
Arm your colon with liquid gold......................214
Say goodbye to stomach pain 215
Stop aging in its tracks 216

Omega-3
Eat your way to lower blood pressure 217
Fish oil keeps cholesterol under control 218
Bone up on omega-3 to avoid osteoporosis 219
Soothe psoriasis with fish oil 220

Onions & leeks
Nip a heart attack in the bud 221
Dodge a very deadly cancer 222
Super strategy for a healthy prostate 223

Onions & leeks *(continued)*
No-sweat way to build stronger bones 225

Passion fruit
Get passionate about stopping heart disease 226
'C' how passion fruit protects your health 228
Melt off pounds painlessly 229
Breathe easy with tropical treatment 230

Peppermint
Soothe your insides with peppermint power 232
Cool remedy for pain 233

Plums
Enjoy a plum-powerful cancer fighter 235
Strong bones deserve proven protection 236

Pomegranate
'Forbidden fruit' cleans out your arteries 239
3 ways pomegranates promote good health 240
Short circuit cavities and wrinkles .242
Powerful pomegranate perks up potency 243

Potatoes
Super spuds save your heart 244
Protect yourself from type 2 diabetes 246
Cut cancer-causing compounds 247
Cold potatoes defeat gut diseases 248

Powdered milk
Cooking trick builds better bones 249
Shore up your body's defenses 251

Probiotics
Boost immunity with beneficial 'bugs' 253
New diabetes fighter protects your heart 256
Relieve IBS symptoms at last 258
Beat stubborn ulcers for good 259
5 ways to sidestep colon cancer 261
Ward off IBD flare-ups 262

Protein
Powerful protection from chicken soup 263
Fight back against weak muscles 264
Melt off pounds the easy way 267
Surprising secret to healthy joints .268

Red grapes

Fruit of the vine protects your heart 270
Sweet path to a better memory 271
Go purple to battle cancer 272
Fight diabetes with a fabulous fruit .274
Stomp out disease-causing bacteria 275

Resistant starch

Little-known nutrient nixes colon cancer 276
Easy way to burn fat and halt hunger 278

Rosemary

Tasty way to preserve your memories 279
Aromatic way to condition your hair 282
3 unusual ways to stay healthy 283

Salba

Chia: secret weapon in heart disease 284

Selenium

Diet secret for strong muscles 288
Simple way to sidestep cancer 289
Keep your joints jumping 291

Soy

Cut through cholesterol confusion 292
Little legume keeps breast cancer at bay 293
Beef up your bones 294
Put the squeeze on lung cancer 296
Get a grip on menopause symptoms 298
Straight talk about soy and memory loss 299

Tomatoes

A double dose of heart protection .301
Delicious secret to smoother skin .302
Hit the 'sauce' for stronger bones .303
New weapon against prostate cancer 304

Vinegar

Tasty way to tame blood sugar 306
Add flavor and subtract cancer risk 307
Fight your odds of a heart attack 309
Clean house without harmful chemicals 310
Meet your indoor-outdoor problem solver 313

Vitamin D

Sunshine vitamin shields you from cancer 315
Revive weak bones and muscles 317

Vitamin D *(continued)*

Surprising way to avoid arthritis 318
Take a bite out of tooth loss 319
Why your eyes need vitamin D 320
Slam the brakes on autoimmune disorders 321
Breathe better with vitamin D 323
Heart disease self-defense 324
Dodge diabetes with a vital vitamin .325

Vitamin E

Guard your heart and blood vessels .326
Dodge the common cold 327
Ultimate vitamin adds vim and vigor 329
Super nutrient saves your hearing 331

Water & electrolytes

Top off your tank for better health .332
3 great reasons to drink more water .334
The latest scoop on low-salt diets 335
Flush out cancer risk 336
Outsmart tooth decay 337
The real truth about 'health' drinks .339

Whole grains

Head off high blood pressure 341
Battle belly fat and win 343
3 ways grains fight heart disease 345
Secret to defeating diabetes 346
Easy way to keep cancer at bay 348

Zinc

Zinc zaps colds and flu 349
Age-proof your eyes 350
Cushion your joints with key mineral 351

Food secrets: More nutrition for less money

Slash your grocery bill 354
Lock in nutrients with careful cooking 355

Index 360

Açai

Rescue your health with the latest 'superfood'

Açai has been getting a lot of attention lately — and with good reason. This little purple berry, pronounced "ah-sigh-ee," is loaded with antioxidants that may protect you from a variety of conditions. Also known as the Amazonian palm berry, the açai berry grows on large palm trees, the same trees that produce hearts of palm. It tastes like a mix of chocolate and berry. Because it does not travel well, it's available mostly in juice or powdered form. Touted as one of the latest "superfoods," the açai berry may actually live up to its considerable hype. Here are some of the ways this tiny purple powerhouse can help you.

Hampers heart disease. Antioxidants come in handy in the fight against heart disease. Low-density lipoprotein (LDL) cholesterol — better known as "bad cholesterol" — becomes a danger to your arteries only after becoming oxidized. If you can prevent that, you can help protect yourself from heart attacks and strokes.

When it comes to antioxidants, nothing beats açai. A system called oxygen radical absorbance capacity (ORAC) measures the antioxidant activity of foods. In a recent study, freeze-dried açai berries posted the highest ORAC score of any fruit or vegetable. Among these antioxidants are anthocyanins, pigments that give açai berries their bright purple color. Anthocyanins are also the secret to red wine's heart-healthy benefits. While açai boasts more anthocyanins than red wine, only about 10 percent of its antioxidant powers come from anthocyanins. That means some other mystery antioxidants are at work within the açai berry. The more, the merrier.

Açai berries also contain potassium and manganese, important minerals that help regulate your blood pressure.

Curtails cancer. Thanks to its antioxidant powers, açai also has anti-cancer potential. Açai's remarkable ability to scavenge harmful free radicals before they can cause DNA damage may shield you from cancer. In fact, açai extract stopped the spread of human leukemia cells by as much as 86 percent in lab tests.

Another study found that, in extremely high concentrations, açai could have mutagenic effects. This means it could cause mutations in an organism, and mutations often lead to cancer. However, it poses a low risk to humans — especially since you're unlikely to consume enough açai to make it dangerous.

Douses inflammation. Like cherries, another fruit rich in antho-cyanins, açai may have a soothing effect on arthritis and gout pain. That's because anthocyanins fight inflammation. Açai has been called a potential cyclooxygenase (COX)-1 and COX-2 inhibitor. That means it could act like ibuprofen and other anti-inflammatory drugs — only without the side effects.

Because inflammation may play a key role in so many conditions — including heart disease, cancer, asthma, diabetes, and digestive disorders — there's no telling how helpful açai can be to your overall health.

Soothes your skin. You don't even have to eat açai berries or drink their juice to benefit from this powerful fruit. An açai facial could help counteract wrinkles, sun damage, and acne. Again, the antioxidants do the trick. Anthocyanins stop free radicals from harming connective tissue. Their anti-inflammatory powers also makes açai an astringent, contracting and tightening skin tissue to battle wrinkles and acne. Açai also contains helpful fatty acids and other nutrients to nourish your skin.

Give açai a try. Look for açai juice in your local grocery store. You may also find açai juice blended with another fruit juice, like raspberry or grape. Other ways to enjoy açai include adding the juice to shakes and smoothies or adding the powder or concentrated capsules to other beverages.

Peach Apple Crisp with Açai Drizzle

Ingredients

20 oz peaches, canned in light syrup and drained

2 med apples, peeled and sliced

1/2 tsp vanilla extract

1/4 tsp ground cinnamon

3/4 cup + 3 Tbs unbleached white flour

1/4 cup brown sugar, packed

3 Tbs margarine, chilled

1 cup açai juice

1/2 cup honey

Instructions

1. Preheat oven to 350°F. Lightly grease 9x9x2-inch casserole dish.
2. Combine peaches, apples, vanilla, and cinnamon in a bowl. Toss well and spread evenly in greased casserole dish.
3. Combine flour and sugar in small bowl. Cut in margarine with two knives until the mixture resembles coarse meal.
4. Sprinkle flour mixture evenly over fruit.
5. Bake until lightly browned and bubbly, about 20 minutes.
6. Combine açai juice and honey, and mix. Drizzle over baked crisp and serve immediately.

(Serves 8)

Nutrition Summary by Serving

225.7 Calories (40.1 calories from fat, 17.78 percent of total); 4.5 g Fats; 1.7 g Protein; 47.6 g Carbohydrates; 0.0 mg Cholesterol; 1.7 g Fiber; 64.8 mg Sodium

Apples

Get to the core of cancer protection

Green, red, or yellow — no matter what color you prefer, apples truly are just as healthy as they're cracked up to be. That apple-a-day you put in your lunch box contains nutrients that are powerful shields against cancer. You'll want to eat your apples whole for the strongest protection.

Queue up for quercetin. Most of an apple's quercetin is in the peel — not the flesh — of the fruit. So wash your apples to remove dirt and pesticides, but don't peel them. That way you won't cut away this important phytochemical.

Quercetin is an antioxidant that stops tumor cell growth. Research hints it may work against cancers of the lung, breast, liver, and colon. A study in Hawaii found people who ate more apples and onions — both high in quercetin — had a lower risk of lung cancer. The well-known Nurses' Health Study, which followed more than 77,000 women, had similar results. Women who ate more fruits and vegetables, especially apples and pears, had less risk of developing lung cancer. But remember — you need to eat the whole apple.

Try for some triterpenoids. Apple peel also stores up natural plant compounds called triterpenoids. Scientists at Cornell University found certain triterpenoids either kill or slow the growth of cancer cells in lab tests. If you like apple juice better than whole apples, stick with cider, also called unfiltered or cloudy apple juice. It's made of shredded whole apples — including the peel.

Pick out some pectin. Pectin, a soluble fiber in apples, citrus fruits, and many other fruits and vegetables, is yet another cancer-fighting ingredient in this tasty fruit. You may know it as a gelling agent for jam and yogurt. One lab study at the University of Georgia found adding pectin to a group of prostate cancer cells caused many of the cells to die — up to 40 percent of them. But pectin didn't kill normal healthy cells. UGA Cancer Center researcher Debra Mohnen believes eating more fruits and vegetables is critical to good health.

"Even though we hear constantly that we're supposed to eat lots of fruits and vegetables, it wasn't until we started working on these studies that it finally hit home how really important that was," she said. "By simply increasing your intake, you're going to get a lot of pectin and all of the other beneficial phytochemicals at the same time."

Snack on the 'super fruit' that's good for your heart

Apples contain a dynamic duo of nutrients to wage a winning battle against high cholesterol and heart disease.

Fill up on flavonoids. These super nutrients help your heart by lowering inflammation and keeping blood platelets from sticking together. In fact, flavonoids in apples — along with other fruits and vegetables, nuts, herbs, and red wine — work as antioxidants. That's good for your heart because they stop the oxidation of LDL cholesterol — the "bad" kind — to protect against hardening of the arteries.

Researchers tested this theory by looking at information from the well-known Iowa Women's Health Study. In this study, experts followed more than 34,000 older women for 16 years, keeping track of what they ate and what illnesses they developed or died from. Women who ate more flavonoid-rich foods, including apples, pears, and red wine, were less likely to die from heart disease during the study.

Reduce with pectin. You've seen it in the oatmeal ads. Soluble fiber like pectin and psyllium husk helps lower cholesterol. It soaks up water in the intestines and forms a gel — a gooey mass that puts the brakes on digestion. Slower digestion of starches and sugars means cholesterol levels go down over time.

Apples are packed with pectin, so a group of scientists decided to test feed ground-up gala apples to rats who were on a high-cholesterol diet. Compared to rats who didn't get apples, those who ate apples every day showed lower triglycerides and raised levels of "good" HDL cholesterol. The researchers think apples may have a similar effect on people.

The experts don't know whether it's the pectin or the flavonoids that benefit your heart most. But you can be your heart's best friend if you get plenty of both from your daily apple.

Want a smaller waistline? Eat an apple every day. Research has found that adults who eat apples and apple products have less abdominal fat as well as lower blood pressure and a reduced risk for developing metabolic syndrome. This set of problems can lead to chronic diseases like diabetes and heart disease.

Bone up on your diet's missing link

What's absent from your diet could be as much of a problem as what's in it. That's the case with boron, a trace mineral that many diets lack. Boron helps you use calcium, magnesium, and vitamin D — all vital for strong bones and joints. Nutrition experts think getting too little boron may put you at greater risk for arthritis.

Osteoarthritis happens when cartilage, the slippery tissue that cushions your joints, starts to break down. That can lead to fluid pockets and misshapen bones around your joints. Pain and stiffness in your joints — most commonly knees, hips, fingers, feet, and spine — mean a lifetime of work and play has taken its toll. Studies show that people who live in places where there is less boron in the soil — and thus also less in plant foods like apples — have a greater risk of arthritis. That makes sense because arthritic bones have less boron than healthy bones.

The good news is you can get an excellent helping of boron in apples and apple juice, which may ease arthritis symptoms. In fact, both healthy treats rank in the top 10 boron sources in a typical American diet. Other favorites with lots of boron include coffee, milk, peanut butter, beans, potatoes, and orange juice. And food sources of boron are best. The form found in plants, calcium fructoborate, is safer and more easily used by the body than boron in supplements.

Pump up the fiber for a great gut

Fabulous fiber is the tough stuff that gives celery its crunch and wheat bread its heartiness. You won't find it in meat and dairy products, so you need to eat plant foods to get this important part of your diet.

Fiber comes in two varieties — soluble and insoluble. Soluble fiber, from oats, barley, bananas, dried beans, and apples, forms a gel in your intestines to move out fatty substances. Think of it like a sponge that soaks up food to keep it moving through your intestines. Insoluble fiber, in wheat bran, brown rice, broccoli — and yes, apples — is sometimes called roughage. It doesn't break down completely during digestion. Instead, it holds on to water and bulks up stool, acting like a broom to sweep food through your intestines quickly. Experts recommend you eat both fiber types, aiming for 25 to 30 grams per day. Both kinds of fiber are important to prevent constipation, defined by doctors as having fewer than three bowel movements in a week.

Apples provide both types of fiber — about two-thirds of it insoluble fiber and one-third soluble fiber in the form of pectin. A whole medium apple scores you about 4 grams of fiber, but remove the peel and it's down to 2 grams. If you're working to increase the amount of fiber you eat, make the change gradually to avoid discomfort.

How about apple juice? People seem to love it, based on how much they drink. Since 1980, apple juice consumption has doubled, while fruit consumption has gone down. But apple juice lacks some of the great things you get in whole apples. One cup of apple juice has only a quarter of a gram of fiber but more sugar than the whole fruit has. It can make diarrhea worse, so avoid apple juice if you tend to have that problem.

An apple a day keeps memory safe

A is for apple and antioxidants. B is for the boron you need for your brain. Put them together and you have a winning way to help protect your memory as you age.

"Ace" your antioxidants. The powerful antioxidants in apples help your brain make more acetylcholine. This neurotransmitter acts like a carrier pigeon, relaying messages to other nerve cells in your brain. People with Alzheimer's disease build up a protein in their brain called beta amyloid, which forms sticky patches on their nerves known as neuritic plaque. High levels of beta amyloid result in less acetylcholine, which means fewer carrier pigeons doing their job.

Acetylcholine plays an important role in memory and learning, so having enough may be the key to fending off Alzheimer's disease. Researchers in Massachusetts studied antioxidants and memory, most recently using lab mice. Some mice in the study drank apple juice concentrate every day, while other mice didn't get the juice. Mice who drank the apple juice had more acetylcholine in their brains and scored better on maze-running memory tests.

To get the same amount of apple concentrate the mice had, you need to eat two or three apples a day or drink two

Pick Red Delicious apples and eat them whole for the best nutrition. Canadian researchers found this variety has the most antioxidants of eight types tested — especially in the peel. But if you must peel your apples, then go for the Northern Spy variety. It has the most antioxidants in flesh alone.

8-ounce glasses of juice. If you prefer a drink, pick cloudy apple juice or cider for more antioxidants.

Boost your boron. The same trace mineral in apples that protects your bones and joints may also keep your brain young. Researchers in North Dakota have been working to find out how boron affects your brain. In one series of studies, older men and women ate either a diet with too little boron or one with plenty. People who didn't get enough boron scored poorly on tests of brain function, including hand-eye coordination, manual dexterity, attention, and memory. You want to keep those skills in your golden years, so don't forget to eat your apples.

Give your lungs a powerful boost

Eating apples at every stage of life may help keep your lungs strong and healthy. Experts think the powerful natural chemicals, or phyto-chemicals, in apples work by reducing inflammation in your airways, leading to less wheezing and asthma.

Researchers around the world have focused on these phytochemicals, especially quercetin, an antioxidant most commonly found in apples and onions. Studies in Finland, Wales, England, the United States, and Singapore all had similar results — eating apples helped people breathe easier. This research looked at more than 83,000 people, including teenagers, middle-aged men and women, and older adults. In every case, people who ate more apples — sometimes five a week or more — had less wheezing, asthma, and bronchitis. There is even new evidence that pregnant women who eat lots of apples may protect their babies from wheezing or developing asthma in childhood.

It's never too late to begin your apple-a-day habit. Some seniors suffer with breathing trouble caused by chronic obstructive pulmonary disease (COPD). That's the technical term for both emphysema and chronic bronchitis, and it's the fourth most common cause of death in the United States. A chronic, congested cough is a symptom of this disease, and apples seem to help prevent it. Experts think the antioxidants in apples help repair lung tissue damage that can lead to COPD. Eat an apple, and breathe easier at any age.

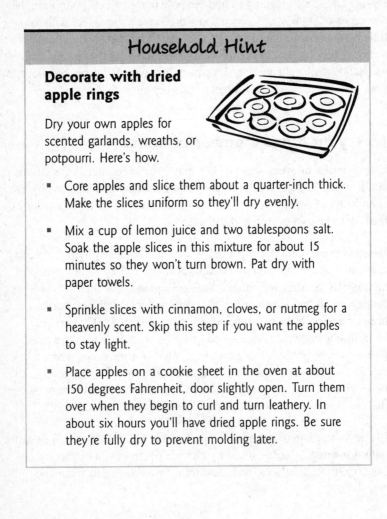

Household Hint

Decorate with dried apple rings

Dry your own apples for scented garlands, wreaths, or potpourri. Here's how.

- Core apples and slice them about a quarter-inch thick. Make the slices uniform so they'll dry evenly.

- Mix a cup of lemon juice and two tablespoons salt. Soak the apple slices in this mixture for about 15 minutes so they won't turn brown. Pat dry with paper towels.

- Sprinkle slices with cinnamon, cloves, or nutmeg for a heavenly scent. Skip this step if you want the apples to stay light.

- Place apples on a cookie sheet in the oven at about 150 degrees Fahrenheit, door slightly open. Turn them over when they begin to curl and turn leathery. In about six hours you'll have dried apple rings. Be sure they're fully dry to prevent molding later.

Aspirin

Save yourself from a hidden stroke threat

Just as too many cooks spoil the broth, too many NSAIDs in your body can cancel each other out. That could erase the stroke protection you thought you were getting from aspirin.

When you take aspirin alone, the salicylic acid in the pill keeps your platelets from clumping together. That, in turn, helps prevent the blood clots that cause ischemic strokes. Research proves it. A recent study found that aspirin taken by itself kept platelets from clumping for up to 96 hours. But when either ibuprofen (Advil) or naproxen (Alleve) were taken with aspirin, that protection dwindled to six hours or less. That could leave you unprotected for 18 hours out of every day.

Oddly enough, this problem may occur because all three painkillers bind cyclooxygenase (COX) enzymes to keep platelets from clumping into clots. If ibuprofen or naproxen get to all the COX enzymes first, aspirin is left out in the cold. So you get temporary clot-preventing ability from ibuprofen or naproxen instead of long-lasting protection from aspirin.

"This interaction between aspirin and ibuprofen or prescription NSAIDs is one of the best-known, but well-kept secrets in stroke medicine," said Francis M. Gengo, lead researcher of the study. Even some doctors may not know about it. So unless you take enteric-coated aspirin, this is what the researchers recommend.

- Take ibuprofen or naproxen at least eight hours before or 30 minutes after taking aspirin.

- Ask your doctor or pharmacist whether you take any aspirin-laced medicines such as Aggrenox. If so, follow the same instructions.

Play it safe: sniff before you swallow

That overwhelming vinegar smell from your aspirin bottle could mean the tablets have "gone bad." Long exposure to moisture breaks down aspirin into acetic acid and salicylic acid. Because acetic acid is the main natural chemical in vinegar, your aspirin smells strongly of vinegar after it expires.

If this happens to you, don't take any of the tablets in the bottle. They probably won't give you pain relief or inflammation-fighting benefits, so throw them out. Also, store your next bottle of aspirin away from damp places like your bathroom. A dry location may help the pills last longer.

Beat cancer at the backyard grill

Get your aspirin bottle ready if you love the tantalizing taste of meat grilled over an open flame. That little white pill may help you avoid breast cancer.

Women who eat flame-broiled or charbroiled foods at least twice a month have 74 percent more risk of breast cancer than those who never eat those foods, a Johns Hopkins University study reported. Eating meat raises your risk to begin with, and grilling them makes the danger even worse. Flame-broiling creates compounds in meats called heterocyclic amines (HCAs.) When you eat charred meat, an enzyme in your body turns HCAs into cancer-causing compounds.

If you are unfortunate enough to have fast-metabolizing enzymes, you will create more active HCAs, which puts you at higher risk for cancer. Women who metabolize more slowly and avoid meat and flame-broiled foods enjoy a lower risk. But surprisingly, aspirin seems to reduce the danger. Researchers found that taking aspirin erased the extra cancer risk in "rapid metabolizers" who ate charbroiled foods. They're not sure why but think it's possible aspirin blocks the activity of the enzymes.

If you do occasionally eat flame-broiled foods or meats, ask your doctor whether you can safely take aspirin with your meal to lower your breast cancer risk. It might be the easiest cancer preventer around.

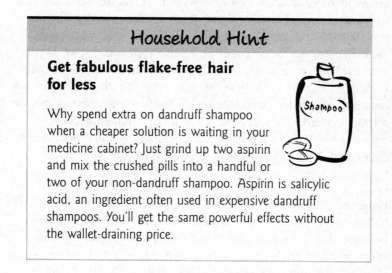

Household Hint

Get fabulous flake-free hair for less

Why spend extra on dandruff shampoo when a cheaper solution is waiting in your medicine cabinet? Just grind up two aspirin and mix the crushed pills into a handful or two of your non-dandruff shampoo. Aspirin is salicylic acid, an ingredient often used in expensive dandruff shampoos. You'll get the same powerful effects without the wallet-draining price.

Aspirin a day keeps 3 health threats away

That aspirin you take every morning for your heart or achy joints has hidden benefits you're going to love.

Shrinks your risk of colon cancer. People with osteoarthritis commonly use nonsteroidal anti-inflammatory drugs (NSAIDs) such as aspirin to help relieve their pain. Because of that, they may be 15 percent less likely to get colon cancer, a recent study discovered. Researchers offer two reasons why aspirin may provide this protection.

- It controls the rapid cell production that is typical of cancer, according to lab and animal studies.

- It prevents the development of colon polyps that can turn into cancer.

Blows away asthma danger. Doctors often uncover new cases of asthma in older adults, which means you're at risk for asthma no matter what your age. Fortunately, the right over-the-counter painkiller may make the difference between developing asthma and avoiding it. Men who took a 325-milligram aspirin every other day were 22 percent less likely to develop asthma, a five-year study reports. Another study hints that those who take acetaminophen may have a higher risk of asthma than people who take aspirin or other painkillers. Although acetaminophen eases your pain, it doesn't fight inflammation like aspirin. That's important because scientists think aspirin's inflammation-fighting power may help prevent asthma from developing in the first place.

Heads off Parkinson's disease. NSAIDs like aspirin may help prevent Parkinson's disease (PD) in the same way. They simply block the inflammation that may trigger the disease. Some experts say damaging events like a severe blow to the head or problems with your genes may cause inflammation in your brain. This inflammation sabotages the cells in your brain that make dopamine, a chemical messenger that carries signals to the brain centers that control movement and coordination. Inflammation may gradually kill off these cells, so your brain makes less and less dopamine. That may reduce motor control in your muscles and cause the tremors and instability of Parkinson's.

Aspirin, ibuprofen, and naproxen fight inflammation by blocking compounds called cyclooxygenase (COX) enzymes. Scientists suspect these COX enzymes may also play a role in causing Parkinson's. But if the painkillers squelch both the enzymes and the inflammation, Parkinson's may never develop. And, in fact, people who took two or more naproxen or ibuprofen pills weekly for at least a month reduced their PD risk by up to 60 percent, researchers report. Women who took two or more aspirin a week reduced their odds of PD by 40 percent, especially if they regularly used aspirin for more than two years.

With benefits like these, that daily aspirin becomes even more important. If your doctor recommends it for a particular condition, don't forget to take it. You may be preventing more than you think.

What every aspirin user should know

Aspirin can cause hearing loss in some, and it may offer no protection from a first heart attack for healthy women under age 65. Talk to your doctor before taking aspirin regularly because it may raise your risk of the following problems.

- dangerous digestive system bleeding

- kidney problems

- stroke caused by bleeding in the brain

- ulcers

- asthma attacks if you already have asthma

Speed up your recovery from knee surgery

Get out of the hospital faster and back on your feet sooner — with aspirin. This little pill could mean a speedier recovery from knee replacement surgery.

Dangerous blood clots are always a risk after this surgery, so doctors prescribe blood-thinning drugs to prevent them. But new research suggests prescription drugs aren't always best. Study participants who received aspirin recovered more quickly and had a shorter hospital stay than people given warfarin or other prescription drugs. But don't start taking aspirin on your own. Some people need a different drug to stay safe, and aspirin may clash dangerously with other drugs you're given during your hospital stay. Check with your doctor on whether aspirin would work in your situation. You could reduce cost, side effects, and recovery time.

Uncover the truth about buffered aspirin

Don't pay extra for aspirin that's labeled "buffered," "enteric-coated," or "safety coated." Although it's supposed to protect your stomach from the damage that can lead to ulcers and other dangers, experts now warn that buffered aspirin may not shield your stomach any better than regular aspirin. Even worse, these pills have a surprise side effect you'll want to know about.

Buffered aspirin's coating does block the release of the pill's stomach-damaging contents until after it passes through your stomach. Unfortunately, once aspirin gets in your bloodstream, it passes through blood vessels in your stomach lining. From there, it blocks the COX-1 enzyme that normally helps protect stomach cells from your stomach's erosive acids — so your risk for ulcers and other problems may go back up.

Even worse, the buffered aspirin coating makes your body absorb aspirin more slowly. That means you may not get aspirin's full pain-numbing impact until three or four hours after you take it.

So don't pay extra for coated aspirin. Instead, talk to your doctor about how you can protect your stomach and — unless he says other-wise — consider buying unbuffered aspirin.

Baking soda

Clear your sinuses without drugs

You can't breathe through your nose, and your sinuses feel like some-one has poured them full of concrete. Nasal congestion from a cold, flu, or allergies can leave you desperate for relief. Try a nose rinse — or nasal irrigation — to breathe easy again.

A nose rinse washes out bacteria and viruses to prevent infection. It also removes pollen, dust, and mucus from your nose so medicine can do its job. All that can cut down on swelling in your sinuses to help you breathe easier. You can get some of these benefits from a nasal spray, but nasal irrigation works better for people with chronic sinus problems. Here's how to do a nose rinse.

■ Mix a quarter teaspoon noniodized salt into 8 ounces of warm water. Iodized salt can be irritating over time.

- Add a quarter teaspoon of baking soda to the mixture. Baking soda acts like a buffer to make the mixture less acidic, blocking the histamine reaction that's so common with chronic sinus inflammation.

- Lean over the sink with your head down. Use a bulb syringe to squirt the solution into one nostril. Hold that nostril shut to keep the solution from running out. Blow your nose a bit, and repeat with the other nostril.

- Throw away any solution you don't use — don't save it for later. Clean the bulb syringe after each use by filling it with hot water, swishing it around in the syringe, then emptying it completely. Place it upside down in a glass to drain.

You may need to repeat the nose rinse several times each day. If you prefer, you can use a special gadget called a neti pot to do the job. You'll find it in most drugstores.

Take the ouch out of bites and stings

Bug bites and bee stings hurt and itch. Find relief in your kitchen cabinet with a baking soda remedy.

For a bee sting, remove the stinger if it's still in your skin. Do this by scraping a credit card across your skin to pull the stinger out. Then make a paste of water and baking soda, and spread it over the injured area. Leave it on for about 30 minutes. Baking soda works because it's alkaline — the opposite of an acid. That means it neutralizes the acid in the bee's venom.

Try a baking soda mouthwash to treat canker sores — those small, white mouth sores that really hurt. Mix a half teaspoon of baking soda in a small glass of water, swish it around your mouth, then spit it out. Baking soda may also block *Streptococcus mutans*, the bacterium that causes cavities.

In a pinch you can substitute a paste of water and meat tenderizer, or simply apply ice to the injury to reduce swelling and redness.

The baking soda home remedy also works on bug bites. For other itchy-skin woes, like poison ivy, chicken pox, or other rashes, try a baking soda bath. Add about half a box of baking soda to your bathtub, and enjoy a soothing soak.

Scrub away food poisoning peril

First it's fresh spinach, then lettuce, and then cantaloupes. Outbreaks of food poisoning from produce contaminated by bacteria have become more common. That's partly because people are eating more fresh fruits and vegetables. It's also because produce often comes from far away and has more chances to pick up bacteria. Make your fresh goodies safe by washing them thoroughly, then storing them in the refrigerator. Here's how.

■ Wash your hands first to keep from spreading germs to other people at your table.

■ Don't use soap on fruits and vegetables. It may have chemicals, and it doesn't work any better than water.

■ Instead, wet your produce, then sprinkle on baking soda and scrub gently with a brush to remove dirt and grime. Rinse thoroughly so you don't taste baking soda. Fill an old shaker can with baking soda and keep it near the sink for convenience.

■ Use lukewarm water — not cold water. The temperature difference between cold water and room temperature produce can send bacteria scurrying. The germs will hide inside your fruits or vegetables, out of your reach.

■ Cut away any bruises, cuts, or damaged parts of the produce, where bacteria can multiply.

3 ways to wash away laundry woes

You can skip those high-priced laundry detergents and pick the cheaper no-name variety. Baking soda helps your laundry come out clean, bright, and fresh-smelling.

- Sprinkle baking soda onto oily stains like spaghetti or pizza. It works as a pretreatment and attacks grease by turning it into soap. Then both soap and stain wash right out.

- Add one-half cup to the laundry along with your regular detergent for cleaner, brighter clothes. Minerals in the baking soda neutralize the wash water to help detergent do its job.

- Deodorize your laundry — just like you deodorize your refrigerator. Freshen those musty towels and smelly gym socks with one-half cup baking soda added during the rinse cycle. Or put some baking soda in the load the next time you use bleach. You can use less so your clothes will be clean and fresh without having that bleachy odor.

Cheap solution for head-to-toe grooming

At less than a dollar a box, baking soda makes for an inexpensive personal-care product to freshen up your whole body.

- Remove hairspray buildup for shining locks. Mix a tablespoon of baking soda into a handful of shampoo, and wash your hair as usual. Don't forget to use conditioner.

- Give plaque and tooth stains the brush off. Baking soda is an ingredient in some kinds of toothpaste, but you can use it straight from the box. Sprinkle it on your wet toothbrush, and brush away the stains. It may be a bit abrasive on your gums, so use care.

- Freshen your breath. The buffering action of baking soda, or sodium bicarbonate, neutralizes odors — even in your mouth. Make a mouthwash with a teaspoon of baking soda in a small glass of water, swish it around your mouth, then spit.

- Soften your skin. Make a paste with three parts baking soda and one part water. Use it as a facial scrub a couple of times a week to remove dead skin cells and leave your face soft as a baby's — well, you know.

- Banish foot odor. Soak your feet for 30 minutes in a solution of two tablespoons baking soda and two quarts water.

Kitchen staple cleans house top to bottom

Baking soda does a lot more than keep odors out of your refrigerator. It's a cheap, natural, nontoxic product that can clean and freshen your whole house. Baking soda gets rid of bad smells with its buffering action. That means it balances acids and bases, bringing them back to a neutral pH. Plus, its gritty texture cleans as well as any store-bought cleanser.

- Safely clean your countertops, bathtub, and other surfaces made of ceramic tile, chrome, steel, and enamel. Simply spoon some dry baking soda onto a clean, damp sponge, then use it like a scouring powder. It will remove dirt and stains without scratching or leaving residue.

- Make your oven sparkle. Sprinkle the bottom of the oven with baking soda, covering all the baked-on mess. Spray it with water several times, then leave it overnight. In the morning, wipe out the baking soda, and rinse away the softened grime. Keep rinsing until the oven shines.

- Deodorize your garbage disposal. Pour one-half cup of baking soda down the drain, then follow that with a cup of vinegar. Wait 15 minutes while the mixture bubbles. Rinse the drain with water and enjoy your fresh-smelling garbage disposal.

- Mix up your own liquid cleaner. Simply stir baking soda into water and let it dissolve, then use it like a soft-scrub soap. You can also add some liquid soap, but prepare it in small batches — it will dry up if you try to store it.

- Do you love the smell of scented cleansers? Make your own sweet-smelling scrubbing powder with baking soda and your favorite essential oil. Start with a 2-pound box of baking soda, then blend in a couple dozen drops of lemon oil, tea tree oil, or peppermint oil. Use a fork to mix it thoroughly.

Cancer early-warning system

Bicarbonate, which is used to make baking soda, could one day help pinpoint cancerous tumors. Your body uses bicarbonate to balance the acid levels in your body. British researchers have found that cancerous tissue turns bicarbonate into carbon dioxide — making the tumor more acidic — and MRI scans can spot the difference. In the future, this may help doctors find very small tumors and also tell them early on if a cancer treatment is working.

Bananas

Lower your blood pressure without pills

Cheery yellow bananas are the tasty, portable snack that adds pizzazz to your cereal and body to your smoothie. They're also a heart-healthy snack with two nutrients to help keep your blood pressure in check.

Potassium cancels out sodium. These two minerals ride a seesaw in your body. If they stay in balance, they help your nerve cells to carry messages, muscle cells to contract, your heart to beat, and so on. But when you eat too much salt, you get extra sodium in your system. That causes your kidneys to pump out more water into the blood, and blood pressure goes up. Over time, that puts more pressure on your heart and blood vessels.

A typical American diet has a ratio of about 1:2 of potassium to sodium. That's way too much salt. Experts say you should aim for closer to a 5:1 ratio, or much more potassium than sodium. In study after study, potassium supplements worked to bring down high blood pressure, but getting it from natural sources is best. Most fruits and vegetables have lots of potassium, and bananas and potatoes are especially high.

Melatonin slashes blood pressure. The other great item bananas bring to the table is melatonin, the sleep hormone that helps your body's internal clock stay on track. Experts already knew people with heart disease and chronic high blood pressure tended to have less melatonin in their systems at night. So they checked to see if taking melatonin supplements might help their high blood pressure.

Researchers in Europe and the United States tested men and women, both with and without high blood pressure. For three weeks, participants took melatonin supplements before bed then had their blood pressure tested while they slept. Both blood pressure numbers — systolic and diastolic — came down during the night after they took melatonin.

Experts warn they don't yet know how melatonin supplements may interact with blood pressure drugs, so you shouldn't put yourself on melatonin supplements if you're being treated for high blood pressure. Instead, get your daily melatonin from bananas, a good natural source of the hormone. Tomatoes, radishes, almonds, and cherries are also good food sources of melatonin.

Shut off your brain for better sleep

Everyone has trouble sleeping sometimes. You toss and turn for hours, while your mind rehashes yesterday's problems and worries about tomorrow's. But sleeping pills are not the answer. They don't work for everyone, and they may do more harm than good. Instead, go natural — go bananas.

Bananas pack a powerful punch when it comes to helping you sleep. First, they have melatonin, the natural hormone that helps regulate your body's sleep clock. Even supplements of melatonin don't always work. That's because the most common dose is 3 milligrams (mg) in the evening, which some researchers say is way too much. It works for a few days, then stops — leaving people thinking melatonin doesn't bring on sleep. Instead, experts recommend a lower dose of 0.3 mg melatonin. Most melatonin pills come in 1 mg or 3 mg doses, so you may be better off getting it naturally from food. You can try herbs like mustard or fennel, but who wants those for a bedtime snack? A medium banana gives you just the right amount of melatonin to help you sleep.

Bananas are also chock-full of carbohydrates to send you off to the Land of Nod. About 93 percent of the calories in a banana come from carbs, making it satisfying and filling so you'll sleep like a baby. Studies show eating carbohydrates before bed helps you fall asleep quickly.

Avoid diabetes with balanced slumber

Getting just the right amount of sleep feels great. It may also help prevent type 2 diabetes.

A study of men in Massachusetts found those who slept about seven hours each night had the least chance of developing type 2 diabetes over 15 years. Those who got five or six hours — and those who got more than eight hours — had a much higher risk of the disease. The scientists think the link may be related to the men's levels of hormones like cortisol and testosterone. So eat a banana or drink some warm milk in the evening — whatever it takes to rest up for good health.

Calm your irritable gut

Cramps, gas, bloating, and diarrhea — or maybe constipation. If these symptoms sound familiar, you may suffer from irritable bowel syndrome (IBS), also called "spastic colon." IBS can bring on abdominal pain and sometimes nausea, headache, and fatigue. There's nothing really wrong with your intestines except for some oversensitivity. Eating the right things can help IBS symptoms.

Bring on the fiber. Doctors often suggest getting more soluble fiber to make bowel movements more regular and lessen IBS woes. A medium banana has about 2.8 grams of fiber, including both the soluble and insoluble forms.

Make room for melatonin. Bananas have another ingredient that may help IBS symptoms — melatonin. This natural sleep hormone is made in both the brain and the intestinal tract, and you can also get it from some foods, including bananas and cherries. Researchers tested whether melatonin supplements could help people with IBS. Eighteen people with IBS took either 3 milligrams of melatonin or a sugar pill every evening for eight weeks. Those who took melatonin felt better — both in their digestive problems and in how they felt overall.

But eating bananas to calm your insides is really nothing new. After all, they're on the menu of the good old BRAT diet — bananas, rice, applesauce, toast — a soothing regimen for diarrhea.

Fresh is best for some fruits

Eat your bananas fast if you want the most antioxidants.

Researchers in Belgium wondered if fruits and vegetables lost their healthy antioxidants as they spoiled. They tested the levels of antioxidants in produce — including broccoli, bananas, spinach, apples, carrots, and grapes — right after they were purchased. Then they stored the fruits and vegetables properly for days or weeks. As the produce started showing signs of going bad, it was tested again for nutrient content.

Most kinds of produce kept about the same antioxidant levels over time, but bananas, broccoli, and spinach lost antioxidants. It's not hard to find fresh bananas. They're harvested every day of the year somewhere in the world. So eat 'em while they're good.

Give your bones royal protection

Calcium is king when it comes to building strong bones and preventing osteoporosis. But it has an entire royal court of nutritional helpers — many of them in bananas.

Good nutrition as you age keeps your bones from getting thinner and weakening to the point that they resemble Swiss cheese. That starts with calcium to keep your bones dense and prevent fractures. You'll also need vitamin D to help you absorb and use calcium, vitamin C to build the collagen that holds together teeth and bones, magnesium to prevent bone thinning, and potassium to help you keep your calcium where it belongs.

Potassium is especially important for older women, who tend to lose more calcium because of modern high-salt diets. One study found women on a high-salt diet who took potassium supplements lost less calcium than those who didn't get the potassium. Those researchers urged women to get potassium from fruits and vegetables in their diets rather than from supplements.

With about 12 percent of the potassium you need every day, a medium banana is a great choice to help keep your bones young and strong. Bananas also bring magnesium and vitamin C to join your royal court of osteoporosis prevention.

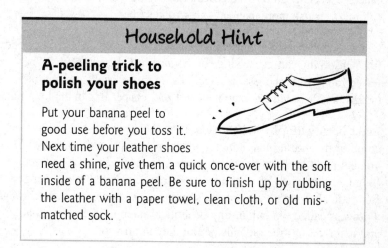

Household Hint

A-peeling trick to polish your shoes

Put your banana peel to good use before you toss it. Next time your leather shoes need a shine, give them a quick once-over with the soft inside of a banana peel. Be sure to finish up by rubbing the leather with a paper towel, clean cloth, or old mismatched sock.

Beans

Fifty-cent food tames cancer

Beans, beans, the magical food ... well, you know the rest. Despite the rhyme, beans are magical in more ways than one. These humble legumes are fast becoming famous, because the more you eat them, the lower your risk of certain cancers.

Fill up on fiber. Sure, lots of foods have fiber — but beans boast more per serving than any other vegetable. In fact, a single serving gives you 20 percent of your daily recommended fiber.

For seven years, Japanese researchers followed more than 43,000 people ages 40 to 79 — a group with high cancer rates who traditionally eat little fiber. The more fiber people ate, the lower their risk of colon cancer, especially among men. Bean fiber came out on top, impacting colon cancer risk more than any other food's fiber.

Lab studies suggest the fiber in beans such as chickpeas keep your body from absorbing cancer-causing compounds called carcinogens. The fewer you absorb, the less damage they do to your cells, tissues, and organs; and less damage may mean a lower cancer risk in the long run.

Fight back with phytochemicals. Beans' cancer-crushing power may come from natural plant compounds known as phytochemicals. When you eat plant foods, these compounds go to work in your body battling bad-boy particles called free radicals. Like rebellious teenagers, free radicals wreak havoc on cells and tissues, damaging them through a process called oxidation. Phytochemicals step in like police, nabbing and neutralizing free radicals before they harm you.

Greek researchers tested extracts from 11 different legumes and found all of them effectively neutralized free radicals. Most also protected cell DNA from oxidative damage, which could be the key to beans' anti-cancer potential.

Beans could especially benefit women at risk of breast cancer. In a study of 90,000 young nurses, those who ate beans or lentils at least twice a week were 24 percent less likely to develop breast cancer. Experts think flavonols, a family of phytochemicals, block free radicals, prevent oxidative damage to your cells, and prompt cancerous cells to die. To aim for the same protection, work at least two servings of beans and lentils into your weekly meals.

Don't ditch all carbs. Cutting carbohydrates has become quite a fad, but think twice if you're concerned about colon cancer. The carbs in beans are a special kind your body can't digest. They end up fermenting in your colon, thanks to bacteria living in your gut. Fermentation produces a compound called butyrate that seems to squash inflammation and abnormal cell growth that can lead to cancer. Plus, indigestible carbs help give beans a low glycemic index. Past research links eating low-GI foods with a lower risk of colon cancer.

Experts recently had a chance to put these theories to work. People who previously had colon polyps removed changed their diets to include more cooked, dry beans. After four years, those who ate the most were a whopping 65 percent less likely to see their polyps return.

You don't need to eat exotic or expensive varieties, either. Thrifty, run-of-the-mill baked, kidney, pinto, lima, and navy beans all cut colon cancer risk. Feasting on red meat regularly has been linked to colon cancer, so consider swapping out a side of beef for a serving of beans once or twice a week.

The more legumes men eat, the less likely they are to get prostate cancer. Three major studies found that eating lots of legumes, including beans, lentils, and split peas, dropped prostate cancer risk between 29 and 38 percent.

Find more folate. Beans are great sources of this basic B vitamin, another weapon in their cancer arsenal. Eating high-folate foods reduces your risk of both pancreatic and colon cancer. Your cells need folate to build and repair DNA. Too little leads to DNA breaks, mutations, and disrepair. Taking folate supplements won't protect you the same way beans and folate-rich foods do, though. So stock up your pantry with lentils, pinto beans, and chickpeas for a dose of natural protection.

Secret to healthy brownies

Brownies can be (almost) healthy. Replacing up to half the shortening in brownies with puréed cannellini beans slashed the fat 40 percent and resulted in fewer calories, a study found. Best of all, beans didn't noticeably change the yummy taste, texture, color, or tenderness of the brownies. This simple substitution can help you battle heart disease and diabetes while still enjoying a treat, plus save you money. Canned white beans cost an incredible 80 percent less than butter and slightly less than margarine, ounce for ounce.

Researchers who conducted this sweet test used canned, cooked beans, then drained and puréed them, replacing half the shortening ounce-for-ounce in the recipe. Out of cannellini? Great Northern white beans should work just as well.

Simple way to sack type 2 diabetes

Bulking up on beans can help you dodge the dangers of type 2 diabetes. This simple food takes on this complex disease in two major ways, without forcing you to cut back on food.

Controls your blood sugar. In general, legumes have low GI values. The Glycemic Index (GI) measures how fast blood sugar rises after eating a food. High-GI foods make your blood sugar rise faster; low-GI foods, like beans, cause a slower, more gradual rise. That's important, because an analysis of 37 studies found diets filled with high-GI foods nearly double the risk of getting type 2 diabetes and make you 25 percent more likely to develop heart disease.

High-GI foods create a spike in your blood sugar, pushing your pancreas to release more insulin. If you're eating mostly high-GI foods, your pancreas is under constant demand to produce more insulin. Like an overworked employee, it can eventually burn out on its job and stop making insulin, leading to diabetes. Sometimes, cells start to ignore the signals insulin gives them to open up and let glucose in. Doctors call this insulin resistance, another path to diabetes.

While high-GI foods increase your risk of insulin resistance and type 2 diabetes, low-GI foods like beans do the opposite. In fact, researchers say these tiny heroes protect against diabetes as well as or better than whole grains and high-fiber diets. Try eating beans in place of white rice, a high-GI food, in dishes.

Keeps you slimmer. Beans may be the single best food for weight loss. One study found that people who eat them regularly weigh less than non-bean-eaters, even though they eat more calories each day.

Great news, especially if you're worried about developing diabetes. Obesity is a major risk factor for this disease. Luckily, beans make you feel full longer and pack a nutritional wallop for a healthier diet. Not only are they slimmer, but people who eat beans also tend to get more fiber, potassium, and magnesium, plus eat less fat and added sugar. A recipe for health, no matter how you slice it.

Half a cup does your heart good

High cholesterol, blood clots, insulin resistance, oxidation — all these factors play a part in heart problems. Beans can battle every one for pennies compared to the price of drugs and supplements.

Head off heart attacks. Just 1/3 cup of black beans a day could slash your heart attack risk almost 40 percent, while eating four servings a week instead of one or none could make you 22 percent less likely to get heart disease. Harvard researchers say beans' power to protect your heart isn't surprising, given their rich stores of nutrients. Their complex carbohydrates lower the glycemic load of meals, while their unique combination of magnesium, copper, fiber, and alpha-linolenic acid boost your insulin sensitivity, help prevent blood clots, and drop your heart attack risk. Plus they're an excellent source of protein, which helps manage your weight.

Belly fat has been linked to heart disease and diabetes. Now, dementia has been added to the mix. A new study shows that having a large waistline and lots of abdominal fat nearly triples your chances of developing dementia. If you're also obese, your risk almost quadruples.

Put the crunch on high cholesterol. Experts say that without a doubt dry beans can improve your cholesterol numbers. Oats may get all the attention, but beans worked just as well in men with high cholesterol. You can probably thank the special phytochemicals in beans called phenols.

Eating half a cup of cooked pinto beans daily for three months lowered both total and LDL cholesterol in people with pre-metabolic syndrome,

Household Hint

Beautify your home with beans

Make table art with leftover dry beans. Find a clear, tall, skinny vase and fill it with different types of beans. Create contrasts by layering colors and sizes, then display it as a striking centerpiece, or use it to hold silk flowers.

a collection of conditions that put you at risk of heart disease and diabetes. Even healthy people can benefit from eating more beans, with a roughly 10 percent drop in their cholesterol, too.

Guard against hardened arteries. These same phenols may also prevent atherosclerosis, otherwise known as hardening of the arteries. Flavonoids, one type of phenol, are natural antioxidants. They disarm free radicals before they can attack cholesterol and oxidize it. That's crucial, because oxidized LDL cholesterol contributes to atherosclerosis. In the laboratory, black beans, lentils, red kidney beans, and pinto beans beat out all other beans in antioxidant power. Not coincidentally, they also kept LDL cholesterol from oxidizing better than other beans. So make them part of your daily diet if you want to watch your numbers drop.

Beta carotene

Heal your heart with a food rainbow

You could rout heart disease, high cholesterol, heart attack, and stroke by loading your plate with colorful foods. Fruits and vegetables come in every color of the rainbow, thanks in large part to beta carotene. It's one of many brightly colored compounds called carotenoids that make foods yellow and orange. It's also responsible for safeguarding your heart.

■ High cholesterol. One of beta carotene's biggest benefits for heart health is its effect on your cholesterol. This nutrient is also an antioxidant, a natural compound that snuffs out dangerous free radicals, much like throwing water on a fire. Free radicals harm your body through oxidative damage. Luckily, antioxidants such as beta carotene keep cholesterol from oxidizing, a process that causes the walls of your arteries to thicken, leading to atherosclerosis.

- Heart disease. Even though many fruits and veggies pack this nutrient, most people still don't get enough. You need around 6 milligrams (mg) of beta carotene daily; most only get 1.5 mg. That's bad news, because deficiencies in vitamins A, C, E, and beta carotene have been linked to heart disease. Build more into your diet, and you could lower your risk.

- Heart attack. Antioxidants from supplements don't seem to protect your heart, but antioxidants in foods do. Evidence suggests eating veggies and fruits rich in carotenoids, including beta carotene, could reduce your risk of heart attack.

- Stroke. Other research suggests two carotenoids in particular — beta carotene and lycopene, which are found in red foods like tomatoes — may put a lid on stroke risk.

Boosting your beta carotene isn't as hard as you think. You won't even have to eat foods you hate as plenty of your favorites are packed with it. Carrots, sweet potatoes, and mangoes are obvious, but some leafy greens contain hidden beta carotene, including spinach, kale, and collards.

To combat these diseases, though, you need to maximize the beta carotene in every meal. The solution is simple — just add a dash of fat. Cook vegetables in a little canola oil, drizzle olive oil over raw salads, or dab some butter on your sweet potato.

Super sources of beta carotene

- ★ pumpkin
- ★ butternut squash
- ★ sweet potato
- ★ apricot
- ★ mango
- ★ orange
- ★ carrot
- ★ tomato
- ★ cantaloupe
- ★ red pepper
- ★ papaya
- ★ watermelon

Cooking, chopping, and grating carrots and other vegetables also helps release beta carotene for easier absorption.

You could eat the healthiest salad piled high with carrots, leafy greens, and other high-carotenoid foods, but if you pour on a fat-free dressing or none at all, you won't absorb any disease-fighting carotenoids. Low-fat dressings have enough fat to help you absorb some, but to get the most beta carotene out of that salad you need to eat at least 6 grams of fat with it.

In fact, add a little bit of fat to the orange, yellow, and leafy green foods you usually eat every day, and you may get all the beta carotene you need without actually changing your diet. Be sure to make smart choices about the kinds of fat you eat, though. Try these super-salad ideas on for size.

- Sprinkle full-fat shredded cheese over salads in lieu of dressing.

- Choose olive oil and balsamic vinegar for a heart-healthy dressing.

- Slice up an avocado or make guacamole to top your salad.

Pumpkins put the squeeze on cancer

Your jack-o-lantern may scare away more than ghosts and goblins. It could ward off cancer. Pumpkins, squash, and other high-beta-carotene foods take a two-prong approach to fighting this disease.

Vitamin A keeps cancer at bay. Vitamin A comes from animal foods such as meat, dairy, and eggs, but your body can turn beta and alpha carotene into vitamin A when needed. Vitamin A, in turn, helps regulate the growth of cells and control immune system reactions. The cells that are affected most by vitamin A live in your digestive tract, in organs like the stomach.

Not coincidentally, eating foods chock-full of vitamin A, alpha carotene, and beta carotene seem to slash stomach cancer risk in half. Swedish adults who got most of

Don't fall prey to diabetes. In a 15-year study, non-smokers with the most carotenoids in their blood were 26 percent less likely to get diabetes or develop insulin resistance. Start boosting your defenses naturally with brightly colored plant foods.

these nutrients from food or supplements were 40 to 60 percent less likely to develop gastric cancer. Other studies show similar results, linking higher levels of vitamin A in your blood to less chance of gastric cancer.

Antioxidants up the ante. Beta carotene may protect against other cancers, too, including esophageal, liver, pancreatic, colon, rectum, prostate, ovarian, and cervical cancers, thanks to its potency as an antioxidant. People with low levels of antioxidants in their diets or their blood stream are more likely to develop certain cancers. By comparison, people who munch on lots of fruits and veggies halve their risk of most cancers.

Stop waiting for the cancer boogeyman to claim you. Start fighting back now with natural sources of beta carotene.

Supplements: a dangerous solution

Beta carotene and vitamin A are good for you when you get them from food or a daily multivitamin, but taking them as individual supplements could be dangerous. Vitamin A supplements may increase your risk of death 16 percent; beta carotene supplements could boost it 7 percent. Those are the results from an analysis of 47 studies involving more than 180,000 people. Also, men taking beta carotene as an individual supplement are more likely to develop fatal prostate cancer, and the supplements seem to raise the risk of lung cancer in smokers.

Vitamin A and its precursor, beta carotene, do a lot of good in your body, but foods are your safest and surest source. Talk to your doctor before you try them as supplements to make sure they're right for you.

Take a bite out of Alzheimer's

You still may not win on Jeopardy, but you'll be more likely to remember where you put your keys if you make a habit of eating foods high in beta carotene. This potent brain protector works in two ways.

- As vitamin A, it normalizes the way your body processes beta-amyloid protein. A breakdown in this process is one culprit behind Alzheimer's disease.

- As an antioxidant, beta carotene seems to boost brain function and brain cell survival as well as improve communication between brain cells. It may also make your brain more resistant to the toxic effects of beta-amyloid buildup in cells. Some research suggests antioxidants, particularly beta carotene, may protect against mental decline in people with the "Alzheimer's gene" APOE 4.

Men who got extra beta carotene regularly for 15 years scored slightly better on tests of brain function than men who didn't, especially on verbal memory tests. Verbal memory scores help predict the risk of dementia. Even though difference in scores was small, researchers say it's important because even small differences significantly affect your dementia risk. In fact, beta carotene worked just as well as the anti-Alzheimer's drug donepezil in studies.

Researchers aren't sure why, but people with higher blood levels of carotenoids tend to have fewer white matter lesions in the brain, which predict the development of Alzheimer's.

Brush the dust off your brain by brushing up on nutritious foods. Bored with the usual beta carotene offerings? Mangoes, papayas, asparagus, winter squash, bok choy, and even packages of frozen, mixed vegetables are all great sources of this brain-saving phytochemical.

Get fitter without moving a muscle

The key to staying independent for the rest of your life could be waiting in the produce aisle. Collards, sweet potatoes, carrots, and kale do more than round out your dinner plate. As top-notch sources of beta carotene, they also help maintain muscle strength and mobility as you age.

Sarcopenia, the loss of muscle mass and strength, makes it much harder for you to get around on your own. It also makes you more frail and increases your chance of falling and hospitalization. But muscle loss isn't just a product of laziness. New evidence suggests the same oxidative damage behind some cancers, heart problems, and lung disease also plays a role. Oxidation damages your muscles' DNA, protein, and fats in a way that may cause muscles to wither with age.

Luckily, carotenoids like beta carotene quench the extra free radicals floating around that otherwise cause oxidation. This, in turn, minimizes muscle and DNA damage. By snuffing out free radicals, beta carotene and other antioxidants soothe inflammation, too. Research links high levels of the inflammatory compound interleukin-6 to sarcopenia, loss of physical function, and even disability.

As a woman, the amount of carotenoid you have in your blood now directly predicts how much interleukin-6 you will have later in life. The lower your carotenoid levels, the higher your interleukin-6 will eventually rise. Low carotenoids also predict muscle weakness and severe walking disability for older women. On the other hand, having lots of beta carotene and other carotenoids in your blood thanks to a diet filled with fruits and vegetables results in better grip, hip, and knee strength in elderly women.

Your carotenoid levels are directly linked to how many fruits and vegetables you eat. In fact, leading experts say eating more of them can help prevent disability in old age. So start munching your way to an independent, active life.

Recipe to fight DNA damage

Oxidative damage builds up in your body with age, but it doesn't have to get the best of you. An intriguing study in the *American Journal of Clinical Nutrition* found that simply eating the right combination of food for 15 days can thwart oxidative DNA damage in older women. According to this research, all you need to eat every day is:

- 1/4 cup of cooked spinach

- 1/3 medium carrot or 1/4 cup of pumpkin

- 1 medium tomato or 3/4 tablespoon of tomato paste

The powerful combo of carotenoids in these foods was enough to protect women's cells from DNA damage. Remember to eat each with a touch of fat to make the most of these compounds.

Potatoes protect peepers from blindness

You can't underestimate the value of your vision. It's absolutely essential to driving, reading, recognizing faces, and staying independent. Unfortunately, the aging process conspires against you with sight-stealing diseases like age-related macular degeneration (AMD). Now, a tiny nutrient can help save your sight and your independence.

Your eye's retina contains millions of cells that sense light and color. The macula sits in the center, allowing you to see fine details and giving you central vision. In AMD, the cells in this fine-vision area shrink or become blocked, sometimes by scar tissue within the eye. You may have only minor vision problems at first, but AMD tends to worsen with age. It's a leading cause of severe, irreversible vision loss in the United States.

Keep your eyesight sharp. Fruits and vegetables crammed with beta carotene helped prevent AMD in studies. One in particular, published in the respected *Journal of the American Medical Association,* found that people over age 55 who ate foods rich in beta carotene along with vitamins C and E slashed their chances of getting AMD by 35 percent.

You can't beat sweet potatoes for beta carotene. Not only do they taste delicious, they also pack more of this nutrient ounce for ounce than any other unfortified food — even more than carrots and pumpkins. It's one of the most powerful foods on the produce aisle. A single, medium sweet potato delivers a whopping 438 percent of your daily vitamin A, in the form of beta carotene. That's not all. This super food gives you 4 grams (g) of fiber, more than a third of your vitamin C, and over one-quarter of the day's manganese, all in a tiny 103 calories with zero fat.

Slow the progress of AMD. There's good news if you already have macular degeneration. The Age-Related Eye Disease Study (AREDS) found a supplement containing a combination of nutrients — 15 mg (milligrams) of beta carotene, 500 mg of vitamin C, 400 IU (International Units) of vitamin E, 80 mg of zinc, and 2 mg of cupric oxide — slashed the risk of the disease worsening by 25 percent. It also slowed the disease's progression in people with intermediate AMD in one or both eyes, or with advanced AMD in only one eye. The next time you go shopping, help your eyes by eyeing the produce department for yellow and orange fruits and vegetables.

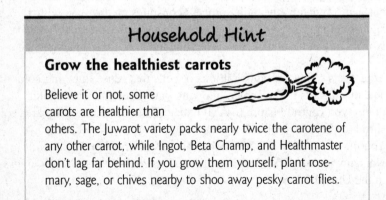

Household Hint

Grow the healthiest carrots

Believe it or not, some carrots are healthier than others. The Juwarot variety packs nearly twice the carotene of any other carrot, while Ingot, Beta Champ, and Healthmaster don't lag far behind. If you grow them yourself, plant rosemary, sage, or chives nearby to shoo away pesky carrot flies.

Breathe easier with beta carotene

"Take a deep breath." Easy enough for your doctor to say, but maybe impossible to do if you suffer from a lung disease. Beta carotene can help. Putting the brakes on lung decline could be as simple as piling your plate high with colorful foods.

Eating more beta carotene foods puts more where you need it, in your lung tissue. There, it helps prevent the kind of oxidative damage that contributes to lung problems like chronic obstructive pulmonary disease (COPD). The connection became starkly clear in a group of more than 500 French people. Those with the most beta carotene in their blood preserved more of their lung function over eight years. Even better, people who raised their beta carotene levels during the study put the brakes on lung function decline.

Carrot juice won't keep unless refrigerated. Keep it cold after you open it, preferably below 40 degrees. Otherwise, it becomes a prime breeding ground for *Clostridium botulinum*, the bacterium that causes botulism.

Natural body processes like breathing actually generate the free radical compounds that cause oxidation. So does smoking. In fact, smoking creates highly concentrated oxidants in your body. Heavy smokers with the least beta carotene or vitamin E, another antioxidant, suffered twice as much decline in lung function as other people and faced a very high risk of COPD.

The take-home message — it's never too late to start eating better, boost your beta carotene, and protect your lungs. Smokers, in particular, need to focus on healthy foods rich in beta carotene and other antioxidants, like spinach, cantaloupe, and sweet red peppers. But don't resort to beta carotene supplements if you smoke. Several studies now show smokers who take these supplements are more — not less — likely to develop lung cancer. Large amounts of beta carotene may block your body from absorbing other anti-cancer nutrients in food, leaving you vulnerable.

Black tea

Enjoy a bonanza for your bones

Milk isn't the only drink that can battle osteoporosis. Tea can boost your bones, too. According to a new study from the University of Western Australia, women who drink tea have significantly higher bone mass density — meaning their bones are tougher and less likely to break easily. The study also suggests that tea drinkers lose bone more slowly than women who don't drink tea.

That's important because your "old bones" aren't really old. In fact, your skeleton is constantly getting rid of old bone and adding new bone in its place. But as you age, your body tends to lose bone faster than it can make new bone cells. As a result, your bones may begin to erode like a crumbling old stone wall. But if you could find something to help you make bone faster, your bones might stay stronger longer. That's how a few daily cups of tea may help. Researchers suspect the flavonoids in tea help stimulate your body to make more bone. In addition, tea contains phytoestrogens like lignans that may also have skeleton-saving powers.

Although some studies suggest the effects of tea may not be strong enough to prevent fractures of the hip or other bones, the Australian researchers found tea to be just as effective as the much-touted combo of calcium and exercise. Other research has suggested that tea may help prevent hip fractures in men and improve bone mass density in older women. So, if you'd like to give tea a try, aim for four cups a day. For best results, make your own "skeleton crew." Combine drinking black tea with extra calcium, vitamin D, and weight-bearing exercises like gardening or walking.

Good news for milk-and-tea drinkers

You love milk in your tea, but you've heard it wipes out the healthy benefits. No need to worry, say scientists from Scotland's University of Aberdeen. Their study found that people who drank tea with milk had no fewer polyphenols and antioxidants in their bloodstreams than when they drank plain tea. So if you've been avoiding tea because you just can't drink it without milk, it's time to grab your teacup again.

More tea means less cancer

Just two cups of black tea a day may help save your skin from cancer. That same two cups might help women avoid ovarian cancer as well.

Defend your skin. Experts say two types of skin cancer — squamous cell carcinoma (SCC) and basal cell carcinoma (BCC) — are on the rise. But now a study from Dartmouth Medical School suggests drinking tea might help prevent both cancers. The researchers found that those who drank two or more cups of green or black tea a day were significantly less likely to develop SCC. Tea drinkers also shaved their risk of BCC more than people who didn't drink tea.

Studies suggest that tea's most potent cancer preventers are polyphenols. Although green tea has more total polyphenols, black tea has its own brand of cancer-fighting polyphenols called theaflavins.

If you want to give your tea even more of a boost, drink it with lemon. The Dartmouth study showed that adding lemon peel to the tea bagged even more cancer protection. An earlier study in Arizona also found that hot black tea with lemon peel helped prevent SCC. People who drank the most tea over the longest period of time seemed to cut their skin cancer risk the most, so indulge as often as you like.

Outsmart ovarian cancer. Those same two cups of tea may have a happy side effect if you're a woman. New York researchers discovered that women who drank two or more cups of black tea daily were 30 percent less likely to get ovarian cancer. The New York researchers think polyphenols are the reason why, but other researchers suggest tea flavonoids like kaempferol and myricetin may lend their powers of protection, too.

5 ways tea fights heart disease

Strokes and heart attacks happen when an artery gets blocked by blood clots, plaque buildup on artery walls, or both. Block one or two of these processes, and a heart attack may simply fail to happen. Fortunately, tea offers five ways to do this.

■ A process called "platelet activation" is a key trigger for blood clots, but a new study from London discovered that six weeks of drinking black tea reduced platelet activation.

■ Stiff arteries coated with plaque are more vulnerable to tears and injury. When this occurs, your body tries to protect the area by forming a blood clot. Studies suggest the natural flavonoids in tea may reduce blood clotting and also make your arteries less stiff.

■ C-reactive protein is a warning sign of inflammation in your arteries — a key trigger for plaque buildup. But research from the University College London suggests tea drinking also reduces levels of C-reactive protein.

■ Plaque buildup in your neck arteries can raise your risk of a disabling stroke, but a French study recently found that women who drank more tea had less plaque in these arteries.

■ Studies have found that flavonoids may prevent the oxidation of the LDL cholesterol in your arteries — another key ingredient in your body's recipe for plaque piles. And a recent Japanese study found that black tea extract may actually lower total cholesterol levels by 9 percent and LDL cholesterol by 12 percent.

In spite of this evidence, other studies on tea and heart disease have been mixed. So the U.S. Food and Drug Administration does not support claims that tea can help reduce your risk of heart attacks and strokes. But while researchers keep looking for answers, it won't hurt to enjoy a few cups of black tea every day.

Better blood pressure by the bag

Lower your blood pressure by drinking tea — and the more the better. An Australian study found that drinking black tea with milk lowered both diastolic and systolic blood pressures in older women. In fact, for every extra cup of tea the women drank each day, they lowered their systolic blood pressure by two points and their diastolic pressure by one point. Those numbers may sound small, but they can have a big impact. If everyone lowered their blood pressure by just two or three points, the researchers say the number of people with high blood pressure would drop by 17 percent, stroke risk would fall by 15 percent, and the odds of heart attack would sink as well.

What's more, you don't even have to drink any caffeine. Experts say tea's polyphenols relax your blood vessel walls and help lower your blood pressure, so decaffeinated tea is all you need.

Drink your stress away

Settle down with a steaming mug of tea after a long, hard day, and you can almost feel that delicious drink draining tension from your muscles and your mind. And, in fact, tea may be more powerful than anyone realized.

Whenever a stressful event occurs, your body churns out hormones like cortisol and adrenalin to prepare you for impending threats. These hormones raise your heart rate and make other dramatic changes to your body so you'll have the extra strength, energy, and alertness to fight or run from danger. But you can't afford to stay in this "red alert" mode for long or your health will suffer. Fortunately, research from the University College London shows how tea can help.

Researchers split 75 young men into two groups. One group drank a black-tea mixture and the other a caffeinated placebo four times a day. After six weeks the participants were put through a series of stressful tasks. Fifty minutes after a task, tea drinkers were more relaxed and had lower levels of cortisol than non-tea drinkers. That means black tea may help speed you out of "red alert" mode and make you more resilient. Stress may still get to you, but you'll bounce back from it more quickly and easily.

The researchers aren't sure which tea ingredients cause this effect, but they say enjoying a cup of tea immediately after a stressful event is probably wise. What's more, drinking four cups of black tea a day may help you handle stress better over the long haul.

New antidote to bio-terrorism

Drinking black tea has many health benefits, but researchers have discovered one that is rather astonishing. A team of Welsh and American scientists found that English Breakfast tea may help defend you against anthrax. "We found that special components in tea such as polyphenols have the ability to inhibit the activity of anthrax quite considerably," said Professor Les Baillie of Cardiff University, the study's lead researcher. Unfortunately, adding milk to the tea erases its anthrax-fighting power so you need to drink your tea black to gain this benefit.

Easy way to combat colds and flu

Drink a few mugs of black tea every day, and you may sidestep more "bugs" during cold and flu season. A small Harvard University study suggests tea may rev up your immune system and help you prevent infections. The researchers believe tea's immune-boosting secret is the compound theanine. Theanine is the trigger for a healthy kind of chain reaction or "domino effect" in your body. That process may work something like this.

- Your liver breaks down theanine into a compound called ethylamine.

- This ethylamine trains your body's first responder team of immune soldiers — the gamma delta T-cells. Like the old Charles Atlas program, ethylamine is supposed to turn average Joe T-cells into muscle-bound heroes.

- When viruses or bacteria try to threaten your body with infection, these improved T-cells race to the scene.

- Once there, they trigger an unusually powerful burst of interferon, a key infection-fighting compound.

- This helps your immune system fight more ferociously against infections, colds, and flu.

But does theanine really have these effects after it turns into ethylamine? Harvard researchers decided to find out. They put one batch of gamma delta T-cells aside while exposing another batch to ethylamine. Then they exposed both batches of gamma delta T-cells to infectious bacteria. The cells that had been exposed to ethylamine produced far more infection-fighting interferon than the unexposed cells. A similar test with blood samples found that cells from people who drank five cups of tea daily for a month produced five times as much interferon. That's why the researchers think tea drinking may protect some people from infection. And even if you still get sick, they say you'll have a milder and shorter case of the bug than someone who doesn't drink tea.

You can drink your tea either hot or cold, but stick with black, green, oolong, or pekoe to reap the benefits of theanine. And don't worry about trying to drink five large mugs a day. Study participants drank five small cups — about 20 ounces — so that should work for you, too.

Nip cavities in the bud

You may love green tea for its health benefits or caffeinated tea for its energy, but if you're prone to cavities, drink decaffeinated black tea more often. It has two special ingredients that may save you money at the dentist's office.

Save your smile with fluoride. Cavities get started when a film of bacteria — called plaque — stays on your teeth too long. Plaque bacteria make acids that erode your teeth and cause cavities. Fortunately, both green and black tea contain the same fluoride as toothpaste. In fact, their leaves accumulate fluoride from the soil the tea plant grows in. But black tea has five times as much fluoride as green tea. And you may get even more if you choose decaffeinated teas because the decaffeination process adds extra fluoride.

That fluoride may help in ways you don't expect. For example, some studies suggest fluoride can counter the tooth-damaging effects of the sugar you add to your tea. Fluoride can also lower the acidity levels on the surface of your teeth so tooth erosion and cavities are less likely. That makes tea a super choice for your choppers.

Add powerful polyphenol protection. Studies suggest the polyphenols in black tea may slash both the number of plaque bacteria in your mouth and the amount of acid they churn out. Add that to the effects of fluoride, and you've got a cavity-blocking defense. Aim for three or four cups of black decaff tea every day for the most protection.

Give hardwood floors a showroom shine

Your dark hardwood floors will sport a rich, gorgeous shine once you learn how to mop them with tea. Here's how. Brew a fresh pot of black tea, let it cool, and pour it into your mop bucket. Dip a microfiber mop in the bucket, wring it out well, and mop a small area. The tannic acid in the tea will make your floor shine like new. Wipe dry and move on to the next section of floor. Soon your friends and family will beg to know how you make your floors look so fabulous.

Blood orange

Go red for great health

Not all oranges are orange. The blood orange gets its name from its bright lava-red juice and pulp. That redness is not just there for good looks. It's a sign of the great nutrients that are unique to blood oranges, making them a great-tasting super fruit. Blood oranges have been around for a long time, but they've only recently been grown in the United States. Before that most came from Italy or Spain. You may find blood oranges labeled by their three major varieties — Moro, Tarocco, and Sanguinello.

Blood oranges may be reddish or even green on the outside — or they may be plain orange. But the inside is dark, ranging from cherry red to purplish. Taste can vary, just like with regular oranges, but it tends to be sweet and less acidic than a "blonde" orange, like a navel or Valencia. Squeeze one for juice, and you get what looks like a cup of blood — hence the name. Blood oranges are so fragrant that their juice is used to make natural perfumes.

Slice into a trio of nutritional goodness. Blood oranges have three phytochemicals — natural plant chemicals — that make them stand apart from other oranges.

- Their striking crimson hue comes from anthocyanins, the substance that gives color to cherries and some other dark red and blue fruits. Anthocyanins are powerful antioxidants believed to slow the growth of cancer cells. Experts think these compounds may work best on cancers of the digestive tract — where they can reach — since not much is absorbed into your blood. Some anthocyanins may also help protect you from macular degeneration, an eye condition that can steal your sight over time. And you can't get them from regular oranges.

- Blood oranges also have naringenin, a natural substance commonly found in grapefruit. Researchers have shown naringenin can repair damage to DNA — the code that tells your cells how to behave — to stop prostate cancer from growing out of control. Naringenin may also help lower your cholesterol, although scientists are still studying that link.

- This newly popular fruit also can boast of a newly found plant chemical — herperidin. It's in the group of phytochemicals called flavonones, and studies on animals show it may lower high blood pressure and high cholesterol. Most of the herperidin is in the peel and pulp, so eating the fruit will benefit you more than just drinking the juice.

Hunt down a rainbow of flavor

Blood oranges and their juice have great health benefits, but they're only available in the United States from about November to May. What's a pioneering chef to do?

You can buy blood orange syrup to use in refreshing drinks, sorbets, and smoothies. Blood orange juice, either bottled or frozen, is available at specialty gourmet shops and ethnic markets. As the fruit becomes more popular, you may find it fresh or juiced at your neighborhood grocery. Buy the juice for drinking or to make vinaigrette dressings, sauces, or pastries. The striking red color will add new punch to your old recipes.

Unfortunately, the same phytochemicals that make this fruit tasty, healthy, and a lovely ruby red cause it to lose some of its good quality once it's juiced, concentrated, and pasteurized. So stock up, squeeze your own juice, and enjoy blood oranges while they're in season.

Put the squeeze on disease. The bottom line on blood oranges is they have fabulously high level of antioxidants, including more vitamin C than regular oranges. That makes them workhorses in the battle against all kinds of health problems related to damaging free radicals, such as heart disease, diabetes, cataracts, and even cancer. And one type of antioxidant in blood oranges — anthocyanins — may behave like COX-2 inhibitor pain drugs, such as celecoxib (Celebrex). That's why anthocyanins battle the inflammation of arthritis and even gout. So juice up your body for health with the tasty goodness of blood oranges.

Chilled Apricot and Blood Orange Salad

Ingredients

8 oz apricots, canned in light syrup, drained and quartered

8 oz pineapple chunks, drained

2 med blood oranges, peeled,
   cut into bite-size pieces

16 oz plain, low-fat yogurt

Instructions

1. Combine all ingredients and gently stir to blend thoroughly.

2. Cover and chill in refrigerator for 24 hours or more.

(Serves 6)

Nutrition Summary by Serving

94.1 Calories (11.1 calories from fat, 11.78 percent of total); 1.2 g Fats; 4.4 g
Protein; 17.4 g Carbohydrates; 4.5 mg Cholesterol; 1.1 g Fiber; 54.8 mg Sodium

Breakfast cereal

Eat breakfast to blast belly fat

How would you like to lose 30 pounds this year? Losing weight isn't
easy. Keeping it off is even harder. But experts say you can do it with
very little effort.

One in five people manages to lose 10 percent of body weight and keep it off for at least one year. More than 4,000 of these successful weight losers participate in the National Weight Control Registry, and scientists are studying them to learn what they do differently from other people. Each has lost at least 30 pounds and kept it off for more than a year.

Turns out, eating breakfast is one of their secrets. Three out of four eat breakfast seven days a week, usually a bowl of cereal and fruit. A few — a mere 4 percent — never eat breakfast. Researchers say successful weight losers are much less likely to skip breakfast than the general public.

They may be on to something. People who eat cereal for breakfast are more likely to have a low body mass index (BMI), a measure of obesity. Women, especially, are 24 percent more likely to have a healthy BMI if they eat breakfast, whereas men who eat breakfast cereal regularly tend to weigh less and are less likely to gain weight as they get older.

The insoluble fiber in Kellogg's All-Bran, FiberOne, and other high-fiber cereals suppresses your appetite, helps you eat less, and improves how your body handles blood sugar after a meal. It helps food move through your small intestine faster, so you absorb less starch. The unabsorbed starch triggers your body to release a "fullness" hormone for two to four hours longer than it normally would. Insoluble fiber also boosts blood levels of another fullness hormone better than low-fiber cereals.

Breakfast-eaters tend to eat less fat during the rest of the day and may choose less energy-dense foods. Plus, they may have more energy for exercise and other physical activities after a nutritious breakfast. They also get more calcium, thanks to the milk in cereal. Getting more dairy calcium is linked to having a lower BMI. Slow down and take time to enjoy breakfast every morning, and you, too, could become a successful weight loser.

A bowl a day keeps diabetes at bay

Experts know eating whole grains can drop your diabetes risk. Now science shows a daily bowl of cereal can, too, thanks largely to cereal's wealth of whole grains and fiber.

People who eat a bowl of cereal seven days a week are 37 percent less likely to get diabetes. Even if you don't eat it every day, having a bowl two to six times a week can still drop your risk 24 percent. Whole-grain cereals offer stronger protection than refined cereals. Here's how experts think cereal works.

Helps maintain a healthy weight. Obesity is one of the biggest factors in whether you get diabetes. High-fiber cereals like those made with whole grains fill your belly so you feel fuller and less hungry, which helps you eat fewer calories. Want more good news? You can eat as much fiber as your body can handle. It has absolutely no calories, and what's more, your body needs it to function at its peak.

Improves insulin sensitivity. Fiber may slow down the absorption of other nutrients, including glucose, in your gut. This helps even out spikes in your insulin and blood sugar that normally follow on the heels of eating carbohydrates.

Experts suspect your cells become more sensitive to insulin over time since you need less of it to handle the more gradual rise in blood sugar. Since insulin resistant people are more likely to develop diabetes, improving your sensitivity may lower your risk. The other upside — less-processed grains have less effect on your blood sugar than refined grains.

Breeds better gut bugs. Eating fiber regularly leads to changes in the types of bacteria living in your gut. It shifts the population from "obese" bacteria — the kind that tend to live in obese people — to "lean" bacteria, which tend to live in slim people. Obese bacteria make a compound called LPS (lipopolysaccharide) shown to boost weight gain, liver fat, and markers of both inflammation and insulin resistance — all factors in the development of diabetes.

Cereal boosts your brain

A daily bowl of cereal could boost your brain health. By helping regulate blood sugar, cereal lowers your risk of Alzheimer's and other dementias.

In people with diabetes, insulin resistance, or chronically high blood sugar, brain cells can't get enough glucose to do their job. This fuel shortage can lead to mental decline in a matter of years. High blood sugar even damages the tiny blood vessels in your brain, contributing to dementia.

High blood sugar also creates damaging substances called advanced glycosylation end products and keeps your body from clearing beta-amyloid out of brain cells. Buildup of both beta-amyloid and these substances are linked to Alzheimer's disease.

You can slash your risk of dementia in three easy steps.

- Eat nutritious foods like whole-grain cereal that help regulate blood sugar.

- Lose weight if you're overweight.

- Exercise 30 minutes a day, five days a week.

$4 secret to preventing heart disease

You could protect yourself from heart failure, coronary artery disease, and high blood pressure for just $4 a week, not to mention start each day with more pep in your step. The secret — have a bowl of whole-grain cereal at every breakfast.

Put the brakes on heart disease. It's the number one killer in the United States. In coronary heart disease (CHD), the arteries that carry blood to your heart become clogged from plaque buildup, a process known as atherosclerosis. As the arteries narrow, your heart can't get enough oxygen and nutrients to work efficiently.

In postmenopausal women with CHD, eating at least 3 grams (g) of cereal fiber daily slowed the progression of atherosclerosis almost as much as treatment with a statin drug. Experts chalk up the benefits to cereal fiber's positive effects on cholesterol, blood sugar, and insulin. Add it all up, and you get serious protection from a food you can eat every day.

Head off heart failure. One in five 40-year-olds are at risk of developing congestive heart failure, a condition where your heart cannot pump enough blood to meet your body's needs. At first, you may feel tired and short of breath after heavy activity, but eventually even light activity may exhaust you. A bowl of cereal every day, however, can make you 29 percent less likely to suffer heart failure compared to those who never eat cereal. It did for men in the 20-year Physician's Health Study. Only whole-grain cereals like bran had this effect, and experts have a few ideas why.

- Cereal-eaters tend to gain less weight with age, possibly because fiber and whole grains help you stay slim.

- Whole-grain cereals pack plenty of nutrients known to lower blood pressure, such as potassium.

- Plant compounds called phytoestrogens in whole grains seem to improve cholesterol levels and insulin sensitivity.

The choice is clear. Next time you go shopping, look for high-fiber cereals with whole-grain ingredients such as bran. Your heart may thank you with a longer life.

Stay sharp at any age

Whole-grain cereals, especially bran, are chock-full of fiber, potassium, and magnesium — nutrients well-known for helping control blood pressure. That's great news, because if you're over 70, high blood pressure (HBP) could be causing mental decline. First, having HBP makes you more likely to develop Alzheimer's disease. Studies link it to the development of the brain plaques, tangles, and brain shrinkage that mark Alzheimer's. Second, HBP doubles your risk of vascular dementia.

The easy fix — eat foods like cereal that help lower your blood pressure. Experts say controlling it as you age may help you preserve your brain power and memories.

Get regular with the right cereal

You've heard the saying, "in one end and out the other." Well, what you put into your mouth makes a big difference in how it comes out. Eating the right foods can ease constipation and keep you regular, with less straining. Here are the reasons why.

First-rate fiber. Bran fiber softens stool, adds bulk, and moves it through the colon faster. Unfortunately, most people fall far short of recommended goals — 21 grams (g) of daily fiber for women and 30 g for men over 50 — but cereal can help you achieve that goal.

Women with pelvic floor disorders who ate a high-fiber cereal every day (14 grams of fiber per one-half cup) improved their constipation and needed fewer laxatives than women who didn't eat the cereal. Experts say straining less during bowel movements can also reduce your risk of uterine prolapse and prevent it from recurring.

Unmatched magnesium. Cereal is no slouch when it comes to magnesium, either. Japanese women who ate diets low in magnesium were most likely to struggle with constipation. Luckily, some bran cereals such as Kellogg's All-Bran and Raisin Bran are great sources of both magnesium and fiber, landing a double whammy in the battle with constipation.

Aiming for more fiber is a good idea, but add it slowly to your diet. Don't bump up your intake all at once. Drink plenty of water as you begin boosting your fiber to help your digestion.

High-fiber diets won't help everyone with constipation. Try it for two to three months and see if your symptoms improve. If not, talk to your doctor about other treatments.

Don't fall for 'health' cereals

Cereal companies are loading their products with yogurt and fruit. Sound healthy? Think again. The yogurt in cereal boasts none of the stuff that makes real yogurt healthy — live bacteria or calcium. Instead, it adds sugar and fat grams. Multi-grain Cheerios, for example, pack more calcium, iron, and nearly every other nutrient than Yogurt-Burst Cheerios, along with less sugar and saturated fat. Similarly, dried fruits may add flavor but few nutrients. Kellogg's Special K Red Berries contains nearly three times the sugar but half the protein and manganese and only one-third the folate, B6, and B12 as regular Special K.

The moral of the story — you're better off buying the regular version of most cereals, pouring on skim or low-fat milk, and slicing your own fresh fruit toppings.

Make-Ahead Warm Rice Cereal

Ingredients

2 cups brown rice, cooked

I cup 1% milk

I tsp ground cinnamon

I cup almonds, chopped

I tsp vanilla extract

3/4 tsp salt

Instructions

1. Combine cooked rice and other ingredients and mix well.

2. Place in a covered bowl in the refrigerator overnight.

3. Warm in the microwave the next morning and serve.

(Serves 4)

Nutrition Summary by Serving

275.7 Calories (121.6 calories from fat, 44.12 percent of total); 13.5 g Fats;
9.6 g Protein; 30.7 g Carbohydrates; 3.1 mg Cholesterol; 4.9 g Fiber;
474.3 mg Sodium

Capsaicin

Cool chronic pain with hot peppers

A plate of hot tamales could be just the thing for arthritis pain, not to
mention backaches, shingles, and diabetic nerve pain. Turns out

capsaicin, the compound in peppers that makes you cry for mercy from their spicy-hot wallop, is a potent painkiller. It's so powerful that drug companies put capsaicin in pain relief rubs such as Zostrix. When you rub capsaicin creams into your skin, your nerves release a chemical known as "substance P" that tells your brain to feel pain.

Every time you apply capsaicin, your nerves release more substance P — but they don't have an endless supply. Eventually, they run out. No more substance P means no more pain in that area. Regularly applying capsaicin cream to one spot can gradually numb joint pain from arthritis and nerve pain from shingles and diabetes. The compound doesn't cure the underlying condition, however. It simply keeps you from hurting.

Capsaicin is not a first line of treatment for most people. It works best alongside other pain relievers or when nothing else works. Experts say it relieves nerve pain (shingles, diabetes) better than muscle pain (back strain, for example). People report relief from hand and knee arthritis as well. These tips can help boost your benefit from capsaicin.

- Wear latex or rubber gloves when applying it so it doesn't get on your hands or in your eyes.

- Rub the cream into your skin until it absorbs completely.

- Leave it on hands for 30 minutes if treating hand arthritis. After that you can wash with warm water if you need to.

- Apply capsaicin three to four times daily for maximum effect. Otherwise, your nerves will restock their stores of substance P.

- Expect arthritis relief after one to two weeks of steady treatment, and neuralgia — or nerve pain — relief after two to four weeks.

Capsaicin may burn and sting when you first apply it, but this sensation fades over time as you deplete substance P. Only about one in three people experience these side effects. See your doctor if the pain persists or gets worse after a month of treatment.

Rub on psoriasis relief

Capsaicin creams may do more than soothe the pain of psoriasis. They may actually help treat it. Applying potent creams containing 0.025 percent capsaicin improved itching, redness, and scaling in people suffering from psoriasis. It may soothe other skin conditions, particularly those with itching, plus ease joint pain from psoriatic arthritis. Talk to your doctor to find out if capsaicin creams are right for you.

Douse the burn of indigestion

Hot peppers sound more likely to cause indigestion than cure it, but these fiery foods may be a remedy in disguise for bloating, pain, heartburn, and ulcers.

Tames your tummy. Hot peppers may cool indigestion the same way they ease arthritis pain — by depleting substance P. Season your meals with red pepper regularly and you'll gradually use up all the substance P in your stomach. Less substance P, less indigestion.

People who took red pepper powder daily in one study felt better after three weeks, with less stomach pain, fullness, and nausea after eating. About half said their symptoms worsened during the first week of treatment then progressively got better, a common pattern with capsaicin. Try seasoning each meal with cayenne or chili powder, and you may see the same benefits. Use one-quarter teaspoon at breakfast, one-half teaspoon at lunch, and another at dinner.

Brings heartburn relief. Common sense may tell you to stay away from chili peppers if you suffer from heartburn, but maybe you should embrace them. Regularly eating hot sauce improved people's heartburn symptoms in one study, because capsaicin depleted their esophagus of substance P. Capsaicin also seems to reduce the amount of acid your stomach secretes. The catch — their heartburn got worse before it got better with this treatment.

Guards against ulcers. Rather than aggravate or even cause ulcers, capsaicin may protect against them. It seems to block anti-inflammatory medicines from damaging your stomach lining. This damage, in turn, can lead to bleeding and stomach ulcers, common side effects from these drugs. Capsaicin seems to protect this lining, possibly by preventing "microbleeding" in the stomach and increasing blood flow to the protective lining.

Contrary to popular belief, experts say eating hot peppers won't worsen hemorrhoid pain or cause ulcers, and aren't hard on your stomach. Some experts do worry that getting lots of capsaicin long term could damage your gut. But others point out that millions of people eat far more hot peppers daily — and get more capsaicin — than the small amounts used in these studies, and without apparent side effects. Always discuss safety concerns with your doctor.

Quench the flames of burning mouth

Swishing your mouth with Tabasco sauce and water could put an end to the misery of burning mouth syndrome. The problem — nerves go a little "crazy," shooting errant pain signals to your brain. Your tongue, lips, or roof of the mouth may burn as if you scalded yourself with hot coffee. Rinsing with Tabasco sauce may help calm those crazy nerves by depleting substance P in your mouth. Swish regularly, and you'll have no substance P to send pain signals to your brain.

Experts also suggest exercising, relaxing, and reducing stress. Medications for anxiety and depression can ease symptoms as well. Talk to your doctor, and get on the road to relief.

Dash of cayenne crushes cancer

Start an affair with spicy foods if you want to ward off cancer. The same eye-watering compound that eases indigestion and arthritis pain may also kick cancer.

Lung cancer. Capsaicin attacks cancer in its Achille's heel — mitochondria, the tiny power generators inside cancer cells. Mitochondria make ATP, the main source of energy in your body. Capsaicin throws a wrench in mitochondria, killing cancerous lung cells without harming healthy ones nearby. It may do the same to pancreatic cancer cells, too. Timothy Bates, one of the researchers at the University of Nottingham who discovered this effect, believes capsaicin could be used to beat cancer. "As these compounds attack the very heart of the tumor cells, we believe that we have in effect discovered a fundamental 'Achilles heel' for all cancers."

Brain cancer. The compound may nix cancerous brain cells, too, according to a recent study. One process healthy cells go through is called terminal differentiation. That means once they develop a specific function, they stop multiplying. Pre-cancerous cells lose the ability to differentiate so they keep multiplying when they're not supposed to. Researchers found that capsaicin helped restore this know-how to abnormal brain cells, which stopped them from becoming cancerous.

Skin cancer. This hot compound squashes a protein known as Bcl-2. When the DNA inside a cell gets damaged, the cell is supposed to "kill" itself so it doesn't reproduce and create more damaged cells. Having too much Bcl-2 keeps the cell from killing itself. Instead of dying, the damaged ones keep spreading. Eventually, this can lead to cancer.

Capsaicin stops cells from over-producing Bcl-2, prompting them to die before they become cancerous and preventing existing cancer cells from spreading. Evidence suggests this process particularly helps prevent melanoma, a deadly form of skin cancer, as well as liver cancer.

Capsaicin's many anti-cancer powers may explain why people living in countries like Mexico and India, who traditionally eat a spicy diet, tend to have lower rates of many cancers that are common in the western world, says Bates. And it may work for you, too. "It's possible that cancer patients or those at risk of developing cancer could be advised to eat a diet which is richer in spicy foods to help treat or prevent the disease," he concludes.

Spicy seasoning melts away pounds

Losing weight could be as easy as turning up the heat in the meals you already eat. Cayenne, chili pepper, banana peppers, jalapenos — they all pack the fiery-hot compound capsaicin. Adding spice to your meals could prevent future weight gain and fight the flab you have.

Experts used to think cayenne and other capsaicin-seasonings could help you eat less. That's true in the short-term. Rats fed red pepper in their food eat less food the first few days but 10 days later are eating their normal amount of food again. The effect on appetite may not last, but capsaicin can still keep you trim and prevent obesity-related illness in three important ways.

■ Boosting the amount of calcium inside young fat cells. Calcium regulates the development of fat cells, and high levels squash their growth. Rats fed high-fat diets with capsaicin added didn't gain weight, whereas rats on high-fat diets without capsaicin became very obese.

■ Putting a lid on the amount of Bcl-2 in cells. The same protein that keeps cancer cells from dying also protects fat cells from the same fate. Capsaicin suppresses Bcl-2 and increases levels of Bax and Bak in cells, two proteins that trigger the death of fat cells.

■ Increasing the amount of adiponectin in fat cells. This chemical protects you against inflammation, atherosclerosis, and diabetes, all obesity-related complications.

Experts say eating a typical Indian or Thai diet, laden with chili pepper spices, should provide you with enough capsaicin to get these benefits. Get adventurous in the kitchen, and start experimenting with exotic, spicy recipes. You have nothing to lose but inches.

Household Hint

Put pepper to work on pests

Hot sauce can make your plants an unsavory snack for insects. Just mix two tablespoons of hot sauce with two drops dishwashing liquid in one quart of water. Pour in a spray bottle, and test squirt on a few leaves. If the test leaves haven't burned after a day or two, spray the entire plant. This homemade bug spray repels big pests, too — it's an excellent deer repellent.

Turn up the heat to beat diabetes

Spicing your life up with hot peppers, cayenne, and other capsaicin-containing seasonings can help turn the tables on diabetes. New evidence shows capsaicin makes your cells more sensitive to insulin and improves the balance between blood sugar and insulin in your body.

The answer lies in inflammation and how the heat of capsaicin cools those flames. Inflammation may play an important role in the development of obesity, insulin resistance, and diabetes. In fact, some diabetes drugs are also anti-inflammatory, and your blood sugar drops as inflammation decreases.

Think of inflammatory compounds as boats floating around your body. They plug into special TRPV1 receptors on some nerve cells, like boats docking in a harbor. This triggers the nerves to release a chemical called CGRP. CGRP causes your body to release more inflammatory compounds, which in turn triggers the release of more CGRP. It's a vicious cycle of disease development, because high levels of CGRP lead to insulin resistance and possibly obesity.

Capsaicin steps in and destroys nerves with TRPV1 docks. This cuts off the production of CGRP, which may prevent insulin resistance and improve glucose tolerance. Capsaicin puts a lid on other inflammatory compounds, too, and boosts levels of adiponectin, a chemical in your body that fights inflammation. By getting inflammation under control, you can dodge insulin resistance, type 2 diabetes, and atherosclerosis.

Start seasoning your food with chili pepper or cayenne. People who added a total of three tablespoons of chili pepper to meals every day evened out insulin and blood sugar spikes after meals. To make this treatment super simple, start each day by measuring out three tablespoons of chili pepper. Use it to season snacks and meals throughout the day.

Cherries

Ease arthritis pain with an everyday fruit

You don't have to pop pills to deal with arthritis. Try a tasty, natural remedy instead. Eating tart cherries can be a sweet way to soothe arthritis pain.

A Michigan State study found that, when it comes to treating arthritis pain and inflammation, tart red cherry juice was 10 times more effective than aspirin — without the side effects typical of nonsteroidal anti-inflammatory drugs (NSAIDs). Anthocyanins, which give cherries their red color, contain anti-inflammatory compounds. That explains why cherries are so effective against inflammatory conditions like arthritis and gout. In fact, cherries decreased C-reactive protein (CRP) and nitric oxide, two markers of inflammation, by 18 to 25 percent in one study.

Long a folk remedy for gout, cherries actually help relieve this painful condition. At the first sign of a flare-up, eat about 20 cherries. You can also opt for dried cherries. Because their nutrients are more concentrated, you need fewer of them to get the same effect. One dried cherry equals about eight fresh ones. If you prefer your cherries in liquid form, here's how to reap the benefits of cherry juice. Mix 2 tablespoons of cherry concentrate with a cup of water. This should give you the power of about 50 to 60 cherries.

Cherries pack a lot of power into a small package. In fact, a 90-calorie cup of Bing cherries contains more antioxidants than a small piece of dark chocolate or 3 ounces of almonds. In addition to anthocyanins, cherries also provide the hormone melatonin, which also fights inflammation and oxidative damage.

You can always find ways to add more cherries to your diet. Just throw some dried cherries into your breakfast cereal, oatmeal, yogurt, salads, and pancakes. You can also add them to couscous, rice pilaf, risotto, and pasta.

Sleep soundly with bedtime snack

Enjoy sweet dreams with tart cherries. Researchers recently discovered that cherries contain melatonin, a natural hormone essential to your body's sleep cycle. As one of the few food sources of melatonin, cherries could act as an antidote to insomnia. Experts say eating a handful of tart cherries before bed may boost melatonin levels and promote a more restful sleep. Melatonin, an antioxidant, may also help you overcome jet lag or adjust to a late-shift work schedule.

Guard your heart with inflammation fighters

Your heart has plenty of reasons to love cherries. Because the anthocyanins in cherries fight inflammation, they may also protect you from heart disease. One sign of inflammation is a substance called C-reactive protein (CRP) — which may be a more important indicator of heart disease risk than high LDL cholesterol.

In a recent study, 18 healthy men and women ate about 45 fresh, pitted Bing cherries a day for 28 days. After 28 days, their blood levels of CRP plummeted by 25 percent. Less CRP in the blood means less inflammation and a lower risk of heart disease. They also had lower levels of nitric oxide, another marker of inflammation.

Cherries also contain potassium, which regulates blood pressure. Other nutrients in cherries, such as vitamin C and fiber, also do wonders for your heart's health.

Little fruit packs a wallop against cancer

Sometimes, big things come in small packages. For instance, you can find several powerful cancer-fighting substances in one little cherry.

- Anthocyanins and cyanidin, two flavonoids found in cherries, have shown promise against colon cancer in animal studies and laboratory studies of human cancer cells. These flavonoids block tumor development and help stop colon cancer cell growth.

- Perillyl alcohol, a phytonutrient found in cherries, thwarts the development and progression of cancer. Studies have found it helps treat or prevent breast, prostate, lung, liver, and skin cancers.

- Ellagic acid and quercetin are other known cancer fighters in cherries, which also provide fiber and vitamin C — key ingredients in any healthy, anti-cancer diet.

Add it all up, and cherries just may provide protection against this dreaded disease.

Chocolate

Tasty treat heads off heart disease

Kuna Indians living on the San Blas islands are some of the poorest people in Panama, but they're the least likely to die from heart disease, diabetes, stroke, or cancer — all thanks to their drinking habit. The island Kuna drink lots of cocoa. In fact, it's their main beverage.

The Kuna living on San Blas grow their own cocoa beans, which are especially rich in flavanols. These plant compounds belong to a larger group called flavonoids. They are a type of polyphenol similar to the ones in green tea.

Scientists noticed that people living on the mainland in Panama were five times more likely to die from heart disease than San Blas Kuna, 15 times more likely to die from cancer, nearly four times as likely to die from diabetes, and an incredible 75 times more likely to die from stroke. At first, experts thought the Kuna possessed an amazing genetic resistance to these diseases, but their true saving grace seems to be all the cocoa they drink.

- Research shows blood vessels function better after eating chocolate or drinking cocoa. Its flavanols stimulate your blood vessels to produce nitric oxide, which helps them work more efficiently.

- Cocoa may even heal damaged blood vessels. People who drank flavanol-rich cocoa three times a day for one week reversed blood vessel damage caused by smoking.

- Cocoa also improves heart and blood vessel function in post-menopausal women with high cholesterol and protects LDL cholesterol from oxidation, a process that leads to hardening of the arteries.

Here's more good news — older adults benefit more from cocoa and chocolate than young ones. Seniors who ate cocoa for several days saw bigger drops in blood pressure and bigger improvements in circulation than young adults who ate the same amounts.

All this sounds great, but the wall of chocolate at the grocery store may leave you wondering what kind to eat to get results like these. Here's a quick guide to help you choose the healthiest chocolates.

Cocoa powder. It makes chocolate chocolatey, packs the most polyphenols, contains little sugar or fat, and boasts an intense chocolate flavor. However, it's not the same as Dutch processed cocoa, which has few polyphenols. Check the baking aisle for cocoa powder labeled "cocoa" or "nonalkalized cocoa." Stir it into water or milk as a bedtime comfort beverage.

Dark chocolate. Because it packs more cocoa than milk or white chocolates, it has more polyphenols. In fact, the less processed the chocolate, the more it contains.

Milk chocolate. It contains lots of sugar but, generally, fewer polyphenols, than dark chocolate. The negative impact on your diabetes risk and dental health may outweigh its heart benefits.

White chocolate. It contains no cocoa and hence no polyphenols, only sugar and fat. A study comparing dark and white chocolate head-to-head found the white had no effect on circulation, while dark chocolate improved it.

Polyphenols don't stay in your body long, so experts say you need to eat chocolate or cocoa regularly to keep the benefits. Luckily, those benefits accumulate over time, so the longer you indulge in a little flavanols-rich chocolate, the more improvement you'll see. Studies don't yet say how much you need to help fight heart disease, but, like most treats, it's best in moderation.

Dark chocolate drops high blood pressure

Indulging in a little dark chocolate need not be a dirty secret. Now you can say it's for "health reasons." The flavanols in chocolate cause your blood vessels to release nitric oxide, a compound that makes them relax. When they dilate and open wider, your blood pressure drops.

One square of dark chocolate daily can bring borderline-high blood pressure back into the normal, healthy range, according to new research published in the distinguished *Journal of the American Medical Association.* Forty-four middle-aged and older adults with mild high blood pressure ate one square of dark chocolate a day for four-and-a-half months. Unlike past studies, this one used regular, over-the-counter dark chocolate you can buy in stores, not special, lab-created, chocolate. Amazingly, store-bought chocolate still brought results. At the start of the study, 86 percent of people suffered with clinical hypertension. By the study's end, only 68 percent did. The others had lowered their blood pressure enough to be in the "normal" range.

Even better, the small amount of dark chocolate people ate only amounted to 30 calories a day, about the same as 1.5 Hershey kisses. Indulging in this little treat didn't lead to weight gain, either.

An analysis of five cocoa studies showed cocoa lowers blood pressure about as well as taking standard drugs such as a beta-blocker or ACE inhibitor. On average, cocoa dropped people's systolic blood pressure 4.7 mm Hg and diastolic pressure 2.8 mm Hg. These changes could lower your stroke risk 20 percent and heart attack risk 10 percent.

People with the highest blood pressure to start with tend to see the biggest drop and the most benefit. Other research suggests seniors have more to gain from a little daily dark chocolate than younger adults. Don't go overboard, but try switching your nightcap with a cup of hot cocoa or that slice of chocolate cake for a square of dark chocolate.

Sweet solution to staying sharp

Lost your keys? Eat a piece of dark chocolate. Cocoa gives aging brains a big boost, probably by increasing blood flow to your gray matter.

In rats, cocoa powder extracts improved their brain function and lengthened their life span. In people, healthy adults who ate flavanol-rich cocoa for five days showed more brain activity while doing thinking tasks. By boosting blood flow to your brain, scientists suspect cocoa flavanols could help slow age-related declines in thinking and brain function, both from normal aging and dementia.

By triggering your blood vessels to release nitric oxide, the flavanols in cocoa relax blood vessels, which in turn improves blood flow to organs and tissue. Nitric oxide also plays a role in regulating the blood supply to your brain. Chocolate could even wake up tired or sleep-deprived brains.

Experts one day hope to use cocoa flavanols to treat dementia, strokes, and other blood vessel problems in the brain. In the meantime, enjoy a nibble of dark chocolate while puzzling out a problem. It just might help.

Household Hint

How to cook with cocoa

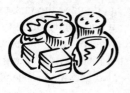

Cocoa presents special challenges that can stump even experienced chefs. These tips will make sure those tears in your eyes are from joy, not frustration.

- Regular and Dutch process cocoa work differently and are not interchangeable. Only use Dutch process cocoa if the recipe specifically calls for it. Otherwise, stick with regular.

- Treat cocoa powder like flour in recipes. If you add more cocoa, subtract that amount from the total flour called for, or the dish will turn out dry.

- To intensify the chocolate flavor, heat the liquid ingredients in a recipe to boiling, if possible, and pour them over the cocoa powder.

- Uncooked egg yolks can cause chocolate mousses and custards to thin. After combining the egg yolks and cocoa, gently heat the mixture to prevent this from happening.

Drink cocoa to look years younger

Get clearer, healthier, younger-looking skin just by sipping a cup of cocoa. You've probably heard that chocolate aggravates skin problems like acne. In fact, it's just the opposite. The flavanols in cocoa can help your skin in two ways.

Provide a smoother appearance. For 12 weeks, a group of women drank a special cocoa rich in flavanols. At the study's end, they had noticeably smoother, more hydrated skin and less scaling. Cocoa flavanols boost blood levels of nitric oxide, which in turn increases blood flow to skin. This feeds more oxygen and nutrients to hungry cells, improving your skin's condition and appearance.

Protect against sun damage. Exposure to the sun's ultraviolet (UV) rays can damage the fats, proteins, and genetic material in your skin, aging it and contributing to skin cancer. Women who drank half a cup of cocoa every day, the equivalent of 3.5 ounces of dark chocolate, boosted their skin's natural defenses against sun damage by 25 percent. They also became less sensitive to UV rays and less likely to burn.

Chocolate busts deadly blood clots

A treat you once thought was taboo may actually reduce your risk of heart attacks for two reasons.

- The flavanols in chocolate and cocoa make your blood vessels release nitric oxide, which keep platelets from sticking together and clumping. This helps stop blood clots from forming.

- Flavonoids, the group of compounds flavanols belong to, seem to help squash inflammation in your body. Research links inflammation to a greater risk of heart attack and hardening of the arteries.

Until recently, studies that pointed to chocolate's anti-platelet effect had only been done in small groups of people, in highly controlled lab environments, and using huge amounts of special, high-flavanol chocolate not sold in stores. Finally, evidence suggests regular, store-bought chocolate has anti-platelet powers, too.

Still, the question remains — how much chocolate do you need to get this effect? Not a lot. Just 6 grams of store-bought chocolate — less than one-fourth of an ounce of dark chocolate — suppressed clotting in one study. Another found 25 g of semi-sweet chocolate chips — less than one-quarter cup — did the trick. Smokers may need more — about 1.5 ounces of dark chocolate daily — to see an anti-platelet effect.

Experts say, given these findings, you can make chocolate part of a heart-healthy diet as long as you choose varieties with less sugar and fat, and eat it in moderation.

Beware of bone thinning

Chocolate may be good for your heart but bad for your bones. This sweet contains oxalates, which keep your body from absorbing calcium, and sugar, which can cause you to lose calcium through urine. Women who ate chocolate daily, in a recent study, had lower bone density than those who rarely indulged. On the other hand, chocolate-lovers weighed less and had a lower BMI.

The bottom line — chocolate may help your heart, skin, brain, and blood pressure, but if you're at risk of osteo-porosis, or if you already have the disease, you may want to cut back on these treats. Weigh your risks and talk to your doctor.

Chocolate Rice Pudding

Ingredients

1 quart 1% milk

2/3 cup white rice, uncooked

1/2 cup sugar

2 oz semi-sweet chocolate morsels

1/2 cup egg substitute

1/2 cup evaporated milk

1/2 cup sugar

1 1/2 Tbsp all-purpose flour

1 tsp vanilla extract

Instructions

1. Place milk, rice, and sugar in large saucepan. Simmer over medium heat; stir continuously.

2. Reduce heat to low; simmer uncovered until rice is tender, about 25 minutes. Check to make sure rice doesn't scorch. Add chocolate and stir until melted.

3. Beat egg substitute, evaporated milk, sugar, flour, and vanilla in medium bowl until smooth. Gradually beat egg mixture into rice mixture.

4. Stir continuously; cook over medium heat until thickened, about 5 to 7 minutes. Do not allow pudding to boil.

5. Pour pudding into medium bowl. Cover and chill.

(Serves 8)

Nutrition Summary by Serving

276.5 Calories (33.3 calories from fat, 12.04 percent of total); 3.7 g Fats; 8.7 g Protein; 52.0 g Carbohydrates; 7.1 mg Cholesterol; 0.5 g Fiber; 100.2 mg Sodium

Cinnamon

Spice up your blood sugar control

You may have heard that a sprinkle of cinnamon is just what you need to keep your blood sugar on an even keel. That's important for people with diabetes, who may have to watch their sweets, eat lots of fiber, and schedule meals carefully for the best blood sugar balance.

Some research shows taking cinnamon supplements could help control blood sugar. In fact, one early study found that people with type 2 diabetes who took as little as half a teaspoon of cinnamon a day lowered their blood sugar by an average of 20 percent. The experts think an antioxidant in cinnamon called methylhydroxy chalcone polymer (MHCP) makes the difference. MHCP seems to behave like insulin to help cells take up glucose like they should. But not all research has proved cinnamon works to lower blood sugar, and experts are trying to find out why. Perhaps variations in the people being studied, like whether or not they were taking diabetes drugs, caused the different results. Some experts now question whether the cinnamon treatment really works.

Another possible problem is the type of cinnamon used in the studies. It was cassia cinnamon, which may contain high levels of coumarin. Eating lots of this natural chemical can cause liver damage. In 2006, the German government issued a warning about overeating a popular cookie — cinnamon stars, which are quite high in cinnamon — because of concern over coumarin.

Too much cinnamon gum, candy, and even toothpaste can cause an allergic reaction. You may experience reddening and soreness of your gums, lips, or tongue. Doctors even saw a case of mouth cancer in a woman who chewed up to five packs of cinnamon gum a day.

It's best to avoid cinnamon supplements, so get your spice in moderation the old-fashioned way. Sprinkle it on your cereal and toast, or swirl a cinnamon stick in your hot tea. But don't use it as an excuse to indulge in cinnamon rolls or similar snacks. A McDonald's cinnamon melt has 460 calories and 32 grams of sugar, while a regular Cinnabon roll has 730 calories and 24 fat grams — not healthy treats for someone with diabetes, or anyone else for that matter.

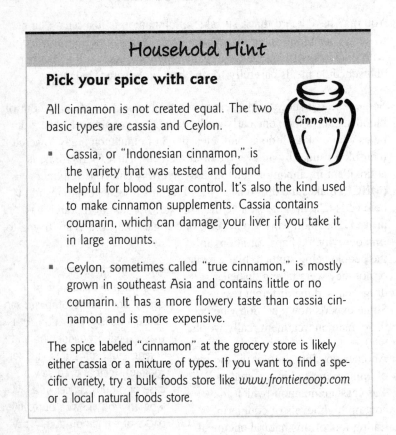

Household Hint

Pick your spice with care

All cinnamon is not created equal. The two basic types are cassia and Ceylon.

- Cassia, or "Indonesian cinnamon," is the variety that was tested and found helpful for blood sugar control. It's also the kind used to make cinnamon supplements. Cassia contains coumarin, which can damage your liver if you take it in large amounts.

- Ceylon, sometimes called "true cinnamon," is mostly grown in southeast Asia and contains little or no coumarin. It has a more flowery taste than cassia cinnamon and is more expensive.

The spice labeled "cinnamon" at the grocery store is likely either cassia or a mixture of types. If you want to find a specific variety, try a bulk foods store like *www.frontiercoop.com* or a local natural foods store.

Heart health: a new reason to season

Get help by the teaspoon for high cholesterol and high blood pressure. A teaspoon of cinnamon, that is. That's because cinnamon is packed with antioxidants and loaded with manganese — both important to keep your heart ticking along happily and your vessels flowing smoothly. Here's how cinnamon works.

Brings down bad cholesterol. You want to keep your "good" HDL cholesterol number high and your "bad" LDL cholesterol number low, and cinnamon may help. A study of 60 people with type 2 diabetes showed taking as little as half a teaspoon of cinnamon every day lowered their levels of LDL, total cholesterol, and triglycerides.

The heaping helping of antioxidants in cinnamon may explain why it's such a powerful cholesterol fighter. Antioxidants in food put a leash on LDL cholesterol, keeping it from oxidizing and doing more damage to your system. You'll get more antioxidant power from a teaspoon of cinnamon than from two cups of red grapes — also antioxidant powerhouses.

Puts a lid on blood pressure. A teaspoon of cinnamon also has about a quarter of your daily requirement of manganese. Don't forget about this trace mineral — it keeps your blood vessels from contracting, which can cause high blood pressure. Researchers tested this idea in the lab, using rats who were fed either a regular or a high-sugar diet. They found that rats on both diets who ate whole cinnamon or cinnamon extract every day had lower blood pressure.

Along with lowering your blood pressure, the manganese in cinnamon may keep your bones strong and safe from osteoporosis. So give your heart and bones a dash of good health.

Scent-sational safety tip

Stay alert and content behind the wheel of your car — even on long trips. Keep the sweet smell of cinnamon in your car in the form of a scented sachet or bundle of potpourri, and you'll be a better driver for longer.

That's what researchers in West Virginia found when they tested how the smells of cinnamon and peppermint affected drivers. Cinnamon helped people stay alert, focus on the road, and avoid being frustrated when things went wrong. Peppermint did all these things, plus it reduced fatigue and anxiety in drivers. If potpourri is not really your bag, try chewing cinnamon or peppermint gum on your next road trip.

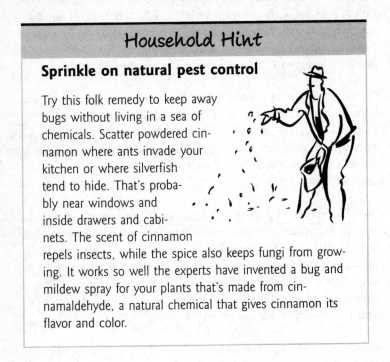

Household Hint

Sprinkle on natural pest control

Try this folk remedy to keep away bugs without living in a sea of chemicals. Scatter powdered cinnamon where ants invade your kitchen or where silverfish tend to hide. That's probably near windows and inside drawers and cabinets. The scent of cinnamon repels insects, while the spice also keeps fungi from growing. It works so well the experts have invented a bug and mildew spray for your plants that's made from cinnamaldehyde, a natural chemical that gives cinnamon its flavor and color.

Citrus

Go orange to save your pearly whites

Citrus fruits are famous for having lots of vitamin C, which battles colds and flu by boosting your immunity, helps your vision, and prevents heart disease and stroke through fighting inflammation.

Vitamin C, or ascorbic acid, is also important to keep your teeth and gums healthy, as old-time British sailors discovered when they voyaged for months with no fresh fruits or vegetables. Their teeth got loose, their gums bled, and many died. They eventually learned to take along the juice of limes and other citrus fruits, earning themselves the nickname "limeys." Turns out the vitamin C in citrus prevented scurvy. People still develop this disease if they don't get enough vitamin C, although developed countries mainly see it in older people who don't eat a variety of foods. It can make your gums bleed, keep wounds from healing, and make you tired and irritable.

Even before any of that happens, lack of vitamin C can speed up gingivitis, or gum disease. That's because vitamin C helps your body produce collagen, which is important for connective tissue like bones and dentin — the part of teeth below the outer enamel. Without enough vitamin C, tiny wounds in your mouth don't heal. That includes damage done by gingivitis, when plaque builds up and causes irritation below your gum line. If the damage gets worse, it can turn into periodontitis — more serious gum disease with pockets of infection that can lead to tooth loss.

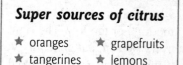

Super sources of citrus

★ oranges   ★ grapefruits
★ tangerines   ★ lemons
★ limes

Research shows that people with gum disease lack vitamin C, but it's not hopeless. In fact, one study found people with periodontitis who ate two grapefruits a day managed to raise their vitamin C levels in just two weeks. They also had less gum bleeding, possibly because vitamin C worked its antioxidant magic to reduce gum inflammation.

It doesn't take a megadose of vitamin C to stave off gum disease. You can cut your risk with just 180 milligrams (mg) a day. That's about what you'll get from drinking two cups of orange juice or eating two oranges, two and one-half grapefruits, or six tangerines. But don't forget you can also get vitamin C from foods like sweet peppers, broccoli, and dark leafy greens.

Smart solution for citrus problem

Fruits are generally healthy for your teeth. They have natural sugars, but they also contain lots of water to dilute the sugar in your mouth. Besides that, eating fruit stimulates the flow of saliva to wash sugars from your teeth. But problems arise from natural acids in citrus fruit like lemons and oranges. They can weaken the enamel of your teeth and cause tooth erosion over time. To prevent that, eat citrus quickly or as part of a meal. That reduces the amount of time acids are on your teeth.

'C' how citrus battles diabetes

Oranges, grapefruit, clementines — oh my. They're all great choices to help keep your type 2 diabetes under control. You need to watch what you eat — and when — so your blood sugar level doesn't get too high or too low. The right diabetes eating plan is different for every person, but generally you should eat a heart-healthy diet; watch your weight; and avoid too much red meat, refined and fried foods, and sweets. Citrus fruits fit into your healthy diet because they have three big ingredients to help keep your blood sugar on an even keel.

Fiber balances blood sugar. Everyone — with or without diabetes — should eat both soluble and insoluble fiber, aiming to get at least 20 to 35 grams daily. Soluble fiber is especially important for people with diabetes because it can help keep blood sugar balanced. Experts think fiber slows digestion and delays the breakdown of carbohydrates so glucose enters your blood more slowly. That means no spike in blood sugar level.

You'll need to eat whole fruit — not just drink juice — to get the most fiber from citrus. A medium orange has about 3 grams of fiber, but orange juice has almost no fiber.

Flavonoids get tough on oxidation. Natural plant chemicals in citrus fruit called flavonoids make it a powerful weapon against inflammation. That's the fancy word for cell damage from free radicals, believed to contribute to many chronic diseases like diabetes.

Researchers in New York wanted to know how orange juice affected people with diabetes, so they tested it alongside sugar water and artificially sweetened water. Orange juice didn't cause more free radicals to build up in their blood, but the sugar water did. So even though orange juice contains natural fruit sugars, it's still a healthy drink for people with diabetes.

Orange juice hasn't always been looked at that way. But some experts say you need to pay attention to a food's glycemic index (GI), or measurement of how fast that food will raise your blood sugar after a meal. Orange juice has a medium GI value, while an orange fits into the low-GI food category. In fact, orange juice can be helpful because it raises your blood sugar if it gets too low. In that case, drink about 4 ounces.

For more information on staying strong and healthy with vitamin C, see the Passion Fruit chapter.

Vitamin C stops stress. Like flavonoids, antioxidant vitamins such as vitamin C wage war against free radicals. But people with type 2 diabetes don't have as much vitamin C in their white blood cells as healthy people do. That's a sign your body is under stress and needs more of this super vitamin.

Researchers found that taking large doses of vitamin C — 1,000 mg a day, a real megadose — may lower blood sugar, LDL cholesterol, and triglycerides. That's great news for people with diabetes, who often have trouble with these health markers. But you'd need to drink 10 cups of orange juice or eat 10 large oranges to get that much. Talk to your doctor about whether a vitamin-C supplement would be helpful for you.

Keep it real for tip-top benefits

Pick fruit or real fruit juice — not supplements or fortified water — to get the health benefits of vitamins and antioxidants found in citrus. Experts say taking megadoses of antioxidant vitamins doesn't really help you live any longer. In fact, too much can be dangerous — even of the "safe" water-soluble vitamins. Taking in excess vitamin C from supplements can cause kidney stones to form.

But getting your vitamins from foods is safe and beneficial. In fact, an Italian study compared the antioxidant powers of orange juice, vitamin C–fortified water, and sugar water. Only orange juice provided antioxidant benefits. This showed it's not just the vitamin alone that helps, but the entire package of fruit or juice.

Cancer cure is no pulp fiction

People who eat more fruits and vegetables are less likely to get cancer. That's the simple truth, shown over and over again. In particular, citrus fruits are a triple threat against cancers all along your digestive tract — mouth, stomach, and colon. That's because they bring three great nutrients to the cancer-busting battle.

Vitamin C curbs cancer. This antioxidant vitamin, so widespread in citrus fruit, battles digestive cancers of many kinds. One study found men who get more vitamin C from food have less risk of mouth cancers, while another found that eating more fruits and vegetables may prevent stomach cancer. Getting vitamin C from supplements doesn't seem to give the same defense.

Vitamin C works by taking the punch out of nitrosamines, cancer-causing compounds made from nitrites in some foods. If there's lots of fat in your stomach, however, vitamin C can't do its job. In that case, it does more harm than good. So make oranges and grapefruits part of a low-fat diet for the best cancer protection.

Limonoids are zesty cleansers. Citrus has about 40 types of these natural plant chemicals, which give the fruits their lovely scent and slightly bitter taste. They help stimulate the enzyme GST to detoxify harmful compounds, turning them into less dangerous water-soluble substances. These are then washed out of your body so tumors don't get started. You'll get the most limonoids from orange, grapefruit, and lemon juices.

Folate finds favor. Citrus — oranges and orange juice in particular — are oozing with this important B vitamin. That's good news since folate may fend off colon cancer, especially in people with a family history of the disease. Experts say folate — or folic acid, the form of the vitamin found in supplements — boosts your body's amino acids to prevent genetic changes that can lead to tumors. Two 8-ounce glasses of orange juice will provide half of your daily folate needs and a good start on colon cancer protection.

Juice up your joint and bone protection

The sunshine fruit does more than just keep your immune system healthy to banish colds. It also contains oodles of antioxidants to defend your joints and bones as you age.

BYO lemon for better health

Think twice before you drop that lemon slice into your water glass the next time you dine out. It may be coated with bacteria.

Researchers in New Jersey tested lemon slices from drinks served in 21 restaurants. Nearly 70 percent of the slices were contaminated with bacteria or yeast — including *E. coli* and other varieties that cause disease. But if you love the lemony flavor in your drink, and you want to get the health benefits of citrus, plan ahead next time you dine out and take your own lemon slice in a sealed baggie. Then you can garnish your own glass.

Add zest to your arthritis battle. Vitamin C and other antioxidants protect your joints by helping you build and repair cartilage. That's the slippery stuff that keeps bones from rubbing together at your joints, but it melts away when you have arthritis. Antioxidants in food also battle the joint inflammation that may be a part of arthritis.

Researchers in Australia figured out that people who eat more fruit and more foods with vitamin C have less chance of developing knee arthritis. That was after 10 years of studying a group of nearly 300 middle-aged adults who ate an average of 218 milligrams (mg) of vitamin C a day. That's more than twice the recommended dietary allowance of 75 mg for women and 90 mg for men. You can get that much from drinking three glasses of orange juice or eating three grapefruits a day.

Support calcium's bone-building efforts. Bones need more than just calcium. They're also hungry for other nutrients like vitamin C to stay strong and avoid turning into Swiss cheese. That's what bone tissue can look like after osteoporosis does its damage. Eat right to sidestep this age-related disease that can steal your height and lead to broken bones.

Eating more fruit may help. In fact, older people who make fruit, vegetables, and cereals the bulk of their diets have denser bones than those who favor meat, baked goodies, or candy. Dense bones means you're not on the path toward osteoporosis. Researchers found that rats who drank orange juice or grapefruit juice every day had denser bones than those who didn't drink juice. They think antioxidants in the fruit juices prevented damage to the rats' bones.

Try some fortified orange juice to get all your bone and joint protection in a single drink. An 8-ounce glass of Tropicana Pure Premium orange juice with added calcium and vitamin D provides 35 percent of the calcium, 25 percent of the vitamin D, and 120 percent of the vitamin C you need every day. That's a lot of bone protection in a single glass.

Household Hint

Treat birds with a fruity, frugal feeder

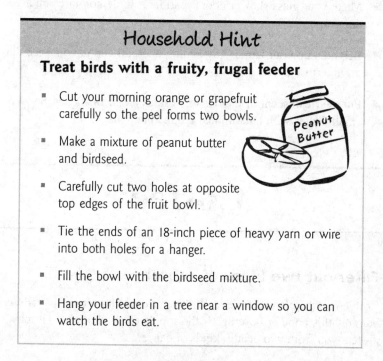

- Cut your morning orange or grapefruit carefully so the peel forms two bowls.

- Make a mixture of peanut butter and birdseed.

- Carefully cut two holes at opposite top edges of the fruit bowl.

- Tie the ends of an 18-inch piece of heavy yarn or wire into both holes for a hanger.

- Fill the bowl with the birdseed mixture.

- Hang your feeder in a tree near a window so you can watch the birds eat.

7 terrific tips for nontoxic cleaning

Clean house without harmful chemicals. Lemon juice — from a bottle or freshly squeezed — does wonders when it comes to making your house sunshiny fresh. Citric acid in the juice gets the credit.

- Toss a lemon slice in the garbage disposal, and flip the switch for a fresh smell.

- Sanitize the dishwasher by pouring a quarter cup of lemon juice in the soap dispenser, then running it through a cycle without dishes.

- Dip a lemon half in baking soda, and remove tarnish from brass and copper.

- Rout out grout from around tile with lemon juice and a toothbrush.

- Make your glass shower doors sparkle using lemon juice on a damp sponge.

- Brighten up your laundry by adding one-half cup lemon juice during the rinse cycle.

- Put the fresh scent of lemons to work as an air freshener. Scatter small dishes with lemon juice around the house.

Coffee

Filter out two kinds of cancer

Coffee may be blamed for everything from heartburn to heart failure, but now this popular beverage is the source of good news — it may protect you from two deadly kinds of cancer.

Escape a silent killer. Liver cancer may be the most dangerous cancer you've never heard of. It usually causes no symptoms until it reaches the most advanced stages. That's why it is more likely to be life-threatening by the time a doctor finds it. Fortunately, coffee may help you avoid this sneaky cancer completely. In a recent review of studies, Italian researchers found that coffee drinkers are 41 percent less likely to develop liver cancer than people who don't drink coffee. Another review from Sweden's Karolinska Institute discovered that liver cancer risk dropped 43 percent when people increased their coffee drinking by two cups a day.

Coffee's cancer fighting punch may come from antioxidants like chlorogenic acid. In fact, coffee is so loaded with antioxidants like these that it's the top source of antioxidants in many people's diets. These coffee antioxidants help prevent cancer-causing compounds from forming and neutralize the free radical molecules that may help cause cancer.

Sidestep a stealthy cancer. Ovarian cancer is like liver cancer in that people with this condition may be symptom-free until the cancer has reached a dangerous stage. But drinking coffee may lower your risk of this cancer as well. In fact, a Harvard study of more than 80,000 women discovered that the more caffeine you drink, the less risk of ovarian cancer you have, particularly if you have never used hormones.

So go ahead and enjoy your daily cups of coffee. Just be careful about how much caffeine you get from other sources, especially if you use acetaminophen (Tylenol). New studies suggest that taking high doses of caffeine and acetaminophen together could damage your liver.

Ward off diabetes with a daily java jolt

The same coffee you drink to wake up in the morning or banish the afternoon doldrums may also help you escape a lifetime of diabetes. A Harvard review of nine studies found that people who drank six to seven cups of coffee a day were 35 percent less likely to get diabetes than people who drank two cups or less. People who drank four to six cups of coffee daily still cut their risk of diabetes by 28 percent.

Coffee may have this effect because it's a rich source of antioxidant polyphenols like chlorogenic acid and phytic acid. Scientists think these compounds may use several tactics to help keep glucose (blood sugar) from building up in your bloodstream.

- They cause your liver to make less glucose to put into your bloodstream.

- They limit the amount of glucose your intestines reabsorb to send back to your bloodstream.

- They help your body resist insulin resistance.

Your cells need glucose for energy, and they often get it from your bloodstream. But cells don't want to let in just anything, so they wait for insulin to tell them when to open up to admit glucose. In pre-diabetes, your cells stop responding when insulin knocks — a condition called insulin resistance. This traps glucose in your bloodstream and allows it to pile up. Fortunately, that's where chlorogenic acid can help. It has compounds called quinidines that help cells respond to insulin so glucose can leave your bloodstream and energize your cells.

Spoon sugar into your coffee, and you may erase its power to fight diabetes. Harvard scientists say their research suggests that adding table sugar to coffee reduces the body's ability to control blood sugar. Adding milk, on the other hand, seems perfectly safe.

But these aren't the only coffee compounds that can help prevent diabetes. Caffeine may have a role to play, too. Some research suggests caffeinated coffee sparks a sharp rise in fat-burning metabolism that may help control your weight. This in turn may lower your risk of diabetes.

Harvard research suggests you may get benefits like these by choosing drip-filtered coffee over other kinds. And the Iowa Women's Health study found that decaff may be better at preventing diabetes than caffeinated coffee. But don't aim for six cups a day. Experts recommend you drink just two or three cups of caffeinated or decaff coffee daily and here's why.

■ A Harvard analysis of women participating in the long-term Nurses Health Study found that two or three cups of coffee each day reduced the risk of diabetes by 42 percent while one cup reduced that risk by 13 percent.

■ A small study at Duke University showed that the equivalent of four cups of caffeinated coffee may push blood sugar levels up by 8 percent.

■ Large amounts of caffeine may interfere with your sleep and could have other unhealthy side effects.

Special coffee boasts super antioxidants

Imagine a coffee that has 10 times as much disease-fighting antioxidant power as wine or tea. That's just what you'll find in torrefacto-roasted coffee, says a Spanish researcher.

Isabel Lopez of the University of Navarre analyzed 11 varieties of coffee and says the fuel behind torrefacto's antioxidant fire is plain old sugar. During the torrefacto roasting process, sugar is added to glaze the coffee beans. Not only does this make the coffee less bitter and acidic, it also creates stupendous amounts of antioxidant compounds. Even after torrefacto beans are mixed with regular beans, you still get extra antioxidants. What's more, Lopez says this coffee doesn't just give you powerful polyphenols. It may also serve up a promising group of antioxidants called "brown compounds" to defend against disease and keep you in the pink of health.

Coffee breaks won't break your heart

Good news for older coffee lovers. Drinking coffee regularly could actually cut your risk of dying from heart disease.

A New York study suggests drinking four or more caffeinated beverages a day cuts the risk of death from heart disease by 53 percent for older adults with normal blood pressure. The added risk of heart attack that commonly occurs after meals may be the reason why. Although everyone has a drop in blood pressure after meals, it becomes more dramatic as you age — a problem that boosts your risk of heart attacks. But caffeine's little surge of energy counteracts this dangerous effect and helps keep you safe.

And that's not the only good news about coffee and heart disease.

■ Drinking several cups of coffee regularly may be less risky than starting to drink coffee or drinking it only occasionally, some studies say. Java may be more likely to trigger a heart attack in people who rarely or never drink coffee, because coffee temporarily raises blood pressure. Studies suggest people who are used to drinking coffee may build up a partial tolerance against this pressure-boosting effect. So new or occasional coffee drinkers may experience a higher rise in blood pressure than veteran coffee drinkers. This extra pressure could dislodge plaque from blood vessel walls, cause artery-clogging blood clots, and trigger heart attacks. Research shows that coffee is less likely to trigger heart failure in heavy coffee drinkers and that one to three cups of coffee daily may actually protect regular coffee drinkers from heart attacks.

■ Caffeine may be less dangerous for your heart if you have the right genes. The way your body handles caffeine depends partly on a gene called CYP1A2. A variant of this gene causes the body to metabolize caffeine more slowly. A recent study found that caffeine only increases the risk of heart attack in people with the variant CYP1A2 gene — not in people with the normal gene. But since you can't be sure which you have, here's the best advice. If you don't drink coffee already, think twice about starting. Not only could it raise your blood pressure, but it may also increase other heart attack risk factors like homocysteine levels and the stiffness of your arteries.

On the other hand, if you regularly drink several cups a day and have normal blood pressure, don't assume you need to give up coffee. In fact, people who replace coffee with colas may raise their heart disease odds by boosting their blood pressure. Harvard's Nurses Health Study found that women who drank four or more colas daily increased their risk of high blood pressure whereas drinking coffee didn't raise that risk at all. Researchers suspect cola compounds called advanced glycation end products (AGEs) may be the reason why colas boosted blood pressure. So check with your doctor before you abandon coffee. This may be one guilty pleasure you're better off keeping.

Beware the kick in decaff coffee

Just three or four cups of decaff from your local coffee house could give you as much caffeine as a Coke Classic. That's what University of Florida researchers discovered when they tested nine decaffeinated coffees from national coffee chains and local coffee shops. On average, each 16-ounce cup contained between 8.6 and 13.9 milligrams of caffeine. Only an instant decaffeinated coffee from Folgers was truly caffeine-free.

Coffee perk: less risk of Alzheimer's

A daily cup of coffee may cut your risk of disabling Alzheimer's disease, especially if you love high-fat, high-cholesterol foods like ice cream. That's because coffee may help protect your brain from dangerous compounds in your bloodstream.

Just as a screen porch keeps pests out while allowing in the sights, sounds, and smells of the outdoors, your brain has the blood-brain barrier (BBB) to keep out bad things like toxins and let in oxygen and nutrients. Even some things that are good for the rest of your body could be dangerous to your brain. One of them — a protein called beta amyloid — may help cause Alzheimer's disease. Researchers think this beta amyloid protein sneaks into your brain through a weakened BBB, where it forms sticky patches of plaque. These may play a role in the symptoms of Alzheimer's.

Unfortunately, it's easy to open the door for beta amyloid plaque. Just eat high-fat, high-cholesterol meals often. Research suggests that could lead to high cholesterol in your blood, which may weaken the blood-brain barrier. In fact, a study from the University of North Dakota recently found that rabbits who had eaten a high-cholesterol diet showed signs of a weakened BBB. But rabbits given a daily dose of caffeine did not. The scientists think caffeine defends this barrier against cholesterol's bad effects. Even better, you may only need one cup of caffeinated coffee a day to do it.

But before you start drinking a daily cup of coffee to prevent Alzheimer's disease, you should know two things.

■ Some studies show that caffeine may help protect against Alzheimer's while others show little or no effect. So don't count on coffee to save you from a faltering memory. Cut the cholesterol in your diet, and take as many other steps as you can to avoid Alzheimer's disease.

■ Be aware that some coffees may contain compounds that help raise your cholesterol. So avoid coffee that's boiled or unfiltered such as espresso or coffees made in a French press. Instead, stick with your favorite filtered brew.

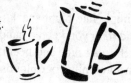
Cornstarch

Bedtime snack balances blood sugar

The same ingredient you add to gravies could end nighttime bouts of low blood sugar. In type 1 diabetes, most bouts of severe hypoglycemia, or low blood sugar, occur at night while sleeping. Getting a grip on these episodes is important, because nighttime hypoglycemia is linked to worsening control over daytime blood sugar.

A simple late-night snack of milk and uncooked, household cornstarch could help you keep a handle on blood sugar. When you add cornstarch to a sauce and heat it, it digests quickly. The sugar in cooked cornstarch hits your bloodstream fast, causing a glucose spike. On the other hand, raw cornstarch — uncooked and straight from the box — digests much more slowly. Its sugar gets absorbed gradually and provides a slow, constant source of glucose for up to seven hours.

That makes it a perfect bedtime remedy to stave off overnight bouts of hypoglycemia. In at least one study, drinking raw cornstarch dissolved in milk before bed reduced the number of hypoglycemic episodes, both during the night and before breakfast the next morning, without any side effects. An added bonus — milk contains tryptophan, a compound that helps you sleep. So a cornstarch-milk drink could not only guard your blood sugar but help you sleep better. Current evidence suggests a 140-pound person should take 4 tablespoons of cornstarch in a glass of milk.

This pantry cure can also help people with type 2 diabetes. A nighttime snack containing uncooked cornstarch helped keep a lid on high, fasting blood sugar, or hyperglycemia, in the overnight hours between dinner and breakfast.

Based on studies, cornstarch works best for people with type 1 diabetes with the following characteristics:

- They tightly control their blood sugar levels. These people are most likely to face bouts of low blood sugar.

- They are "hypoglycemic unaware," that is, do not recognize warning signs of low blood sugar.

- They exercise. Raw cornstarch before exercising can help keep blood sugar from crashing afterward.

- They drink alcohol. Taking uncooked cornstarch after drinking alcohol may help dodge the dip in blood sugar.

Cornstarch works as a preventive measure against low blood sugar, but don't use it to treat existing hypoglycemia. It simply doesn't digest quickly enough to rescue you from a dangerous bout of low blood sugar.

Simple swaps for missing ingredients

Running out of a crucial ingredient doesn't have to ruin your recipe. As long as you have these basics on hand, you can save your meal.

Missing ingredient	Suitable substitute
Baking powder, double-acting	1/4 tsp baking soda plus 1/2 tsp cream of tartar and 1/4 tsp cornstarch for 1 tsp baking powder
Whole egg	1 Tbsp cornstarch for up to one of every three eggs in baking; add more liquid if necessary
Confectioner's or powdered sugar	1 cup granulated sugar plus 1 Tbsp cornstarch; process in food processor until powdery
All-purpose flour (for thickening)	1/2 Tbsp cornstarch for 1 Tbsp flour
All-purpose flour (for baking)	1/2 cup cornstarch plus 1/2 cup rye, potato, or rice flour for 1 cup all-purpose flour
Arrowroot for thickening	1 Tbsp cornstarch for 1 Tbsp arrowroot

Soothe skin with silky solution

Cornstarch does more than thicken sauces. It's great for soothing dry, sunburned, and irritated skin as well as protecting skin from the ravages of chemotherapy.

Relieve dry skin. Make a paste from two cups of cornstarch and four cups of water. Boil the mixture then pour into a half-full bathtub. Be careful, as it will make the bath slippery.

Heal hives. Climb into a soothing bath with six tablespoons of oatmeal and three tablespoons of cornstarch added. Some people say cornstarch baths ease poison ivy itching, too. Try adding a box of baking soda and one and a half cups of cornstarch to bath water, then soak.

Soothe sunburns. Dissolve a half to one cup of cornstarch in a bath of cool water and soak. You can also make a paste of cornstarch and water and apply directly to your sunburn.

Calm cancer itching. Radiation therapy for cancer can seriously dry out your skin, because it kills skin cells and the oily glands in your skin that keep it hydrated. You can protect your skin by dusting itchy, irradiated areas with cornstarch after bathing.

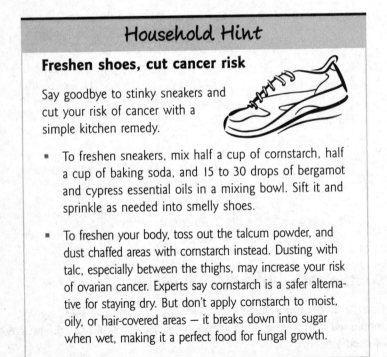

Household Hint

Freshen shoes, cut cancer risk

Say goodbye to stinky sneakers and cut your risk of cancer with a simple kitchen remedy.

- To freshen sneakers, mix half a cup of cornstarch, half a cup of baking soda, and 15 to 30 drops of bergamot and cypress essential oils in a mixing bowl. Sift it and sprinkle as needed into smelly shoes.

- To freshen your body, toss out the talcum powder, and dust chaffed areas with cornstarch instead. Dusting with talc, especially between the thighs, may increase your risk of ovarian cancer. Experts say cornstarch is a safer alternative for staying dry. But don't apply cornstarch to moist, oily, or hair-covered areas — it breaks down into sugar when wet, making it a perfect food for fungal growth.

Cranberries

Wash away bacteria for all-over health

Cranberries have natural chemicals that keep harmful bacteria from getting a foothold in your system. That may keep you free of infections in your mouth, stomach, and urinary tract.

Steer clear of UTIs. Most women get a urinary tract infection (UTI) on occasion, and some get them over and over. Drinking cranberry juice is a common folk remedy when you have pain, burning, and the need to go and go. Science proves it may work to prevent these pesky infections.

People used to think the acidity in cranberry juice made your bladder an unwelcome place for bacteria to live. Now experts believe natural plant chemicals called proanthocyanidins (PACs) in cranberries should get the credit. These PACs keep bacteria from clinging to the walls of your urinary tract, stopping an infection in its tracks. Drinking cranberry juice may also help you get over an infection once it starts.

You can get the same effect from eating dried sweetened cranberries, a tasty snack similar to raisins. If you like the traditional remedy, try to drink at least one or two cups of cranberry juice a day to prevent UTIs. It also acts as a natural diuretic to get rid of extra water from your body and cut down on swelling.

Guard against stomach ulcers. Another body part reaps the same benefit. Natural plant chemicals in cranberries also keep *H. pylori* bacteria from grabbing hold in your stomach. Bacteria — not stress or bad eating habits — are to blame for most stomach ulcers. And infection by *H. pylori* causes other problems, including acid reflux and stomach cancer. A study in China found that people who drank about two cups of cranberry juice every day cut their risk of *H. pylori* infection in just three months.

Avoid dental plaque. You may have seen dental floss and toothpaste made with cranberry extracts. That's because cranberries may also keep mouth bacteria from forming plaque, the first step to cavities. Lab studies have shown cranberry juice can keep *S. mutans,* the bacteria responsible for plaque, from sticking to surfaces. Slow down plaque, and you may also slow down gum disease. But as with other fruit juices with natural sugars and acids, it's best to drink your cranberry juice all at once. Sipping it slowly all day allows the juice to eat away at your teeth.

Cranberry benefits at a glance

You don't have to eat whole cranberries to get their health benefits, but form does make a difference. Whole berries have the most fiber in a serving, but cranberry juice cocktail has the most vitamin C because it's fortified during processing.

Nutrient	Whole raw berries (1 cup)	Dried sweetened berries (1/3 cup)	Unsweetened juice (1 cup)	Juice (27%) cocktail (1 cup)
Calories	44	123	116	137
Fiber (grams)	4.4	2.3	0.3	0
Potassium (mg)	81	16	194	35
Vitamin C (mg)	12.6	0.1	23.6	107
Vitamin E (mg)	1.14	0.43	3.04	0.56
Beta carotene (mcg)	34.2	0	68.3	13

Little red berry offers triple defense

Drink a glass of cranberry juice every morning, and you'll help protect your heart. In fact, the American Heart Association calls some cranberry products "heart healthy" because of their fabulous nutrients. These crimson cuties can help in three big ways.

Beat down bad cholesterol. Flavonoids, natural plant chemicals in cranberries, slow the oxidation of "bad" LDL cholesterol. Research shows this means cranberries can lower your cholesterol and prevent dangerous inflammation, which may lead to heart disease. One cup of cranberries has the same antioxidant power to lower LDL as 1,000 milligrams of vitamin C. That's a lot of armor in a small package.

White cranberry juice gives you all the health benefits of red juice, yet it won't stain your carpet. It's made from typical cranberries that are mature, but not fully ripe. They don't take on their lovely scarlet color until the final few weeks of growth. It's also less tart than red juice.

Pump up good cholesterol. You can think of "good" HDL cholesterol as the opposite of LDL — it whisks away bad cholesterol from your arteries to your liver and then out of your body. That's why a higher HDL number is better. Experts say drinking cranberry juice can raise your HDL cholesterol. One study found that men who drank as little as 8 ounces a day had higher HDL and better heart protection.

Send your arteries to yoga class. Relaxed blood vessels are wide open, letting blood flow through with little pressure. Polyphenols and flavonoids in cranberries make your arteries more flexible so your blood pressure stays low. As an added bonus, cranberries help your body absorb aspirin better. That may give a real boost to your daily aspirin therapy.

Tell food bacteria to take a hike

Cranberry sauce can give your meal more than just good flavor. It may keep food poisoning from spoiling the fun. That's because cranberries put a stop to food contamination by blocking the most common bacteria. That includes *E. coli, Listeria,* and *Salmonella,* which can taint meat and seafood. Mix in some oregano for even more protection. Scientists found that the combination proved to be a potent antibacterial force when tested on beef and fish.

Berry breakthrough in cancer battle

The fruit of the bog may turn out to be an ideal natural treatment for cancer. That's because cranberries are packed with natural plant chemicals that help fight and even treat cancer.

"There are so many compounds in cranberries capable of having some anti-cancer mechanism that when taken together there is potential for benefit," says researcher Catherine Neto from the University of Massachusetts–Dartmouth. "Anti-cancer activity has been reported in the literature from way back."

■ Cancer-fighting ingredients in cranberries include quercetin, which is also plentiful in apples and onions. This phytochemical causes cancer cells to die before they have a chance to do much damage.

■ Another heavy hitter is ursolic acid, found in cranberry peel. It keeps cancer cells from growing out of control.

- A third powerful protector is something called proanthocyanidins (PACs). These natural substances block cancer cells from growing and migrating to other parts of your body. That may keep tumors from spreading.

PACs also make ovarian cancer cells more sensitive to platinum-type chemotherapy. That's a huge plus, because cancer cells sometimes become resistant to chemo drugs. When doctors have to use higher chemo doses, patients can suffer from bad side effects. Researchers found this benefit using the equivalent of just one cup of cranberry juice.

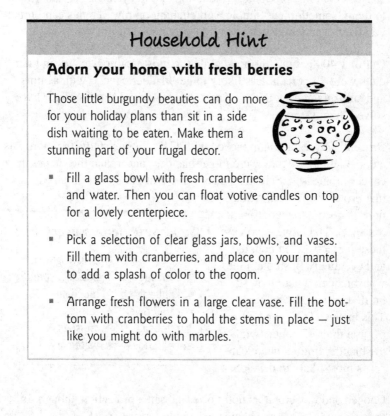

Household Hint

Adorn your home with fresh berries

Those little burgundy beauties can do more for your holiday plans than sit in a side dish waiting to be eaten. Make them a stunning part of your frugal decor.

- Fill a glass bowl with fresh cranberries and water. Then you can float votive candles on top for a lovely centerpiece.

- Pick a selection of clear glass jars, bowls, and vases. Fill them with cranberries, and place on your mantel to add a splash of color to the room.

- Arrange fresh flowers in a large clear vase. Fill the bottom with cranberries to hold the stems in place — just like you might do with marbles.

Cruciferous vegetables

Tender sprouts safeguard bladder

Cruciferous vegetables like broccoli, cabbage, and kale pack lots of cancer-crushing compounds, including isothiocyanates (ITCs). Thanks to them, something as simple as munching on raw veggies can protect you from bladder cancer.

Out of 1,400 people, those who ate the most isothiocyanates in their diets were 29 percent less likely to get bladder cancer, with seniors and smokers getting the most protection. Animal studies might have solved the mystery.

Broccoli sprouts are jam-packed with ITCs. In one study, the more rats ate, the less likely they were to get bladder cancer, and the slower the cancer progressed. Scientists discovered that ITCs boosted enzymes that protect cells from oxidation, a process that contributes to cancer. The kidneys process these protective compounds and eventually flush them into your bladder, where they sit until you go to the bathroom. This means ITCs spend a lot of time in close contact with the bladder lining, where cancer is most likely to develop.

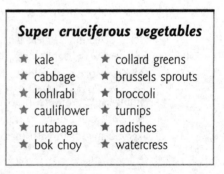

Super cruciferous vegetables

- ★ kale
- ★ cabbage
- ★ kohlrabi
- ★ cauliflower
- ★ rutabaga
- ★ bok choy
- ★ collard greens
- ★ brussels sprouts
- ★ broccoli
- ★ turnips
- ★ radishes
- ★ watercress

Cooked and raw crucifers don't offer the same protection, though. In another study only raw veggies seemed to lower the risk of this disease, and people needed to eat three or more servings each month to gain protection. Cooking can destroy the isothiocyanates in cruciferous vegetables like cauliflower. So break out the raw veggie tray for your visitors, whip up fresh cole slaw, and munch on fresh broccoli when you need a quick snack.

Super 'sunscreen' stops skin cancer

Slathering on a broccoli skin cream could be the next step in sun protection.

Rubbing on an extract made from broccoli sprouts protected people's skin cells from UV sun damage, the kind that leads to sunburns and skin cancer. The secret ingredient — sulforaphane, a plant compound in broccoli. Unlike sunscreen, this broccoli cream did not block or absorb UV rays. Instead, it revved up the body's natural defenses, activating enzymes that neutralize sun damage in skin cells. It also lasted longer than sunscreen, protecting skin for up to three days. Experts say it won't interfere with your skin's ability to make vitamin D, either, the way sunscreen does.

The cream isn't available for sale yet, but until then, keep eating those crucifers. They just might "rub off" on you.

Beat the odds against breast cancer

A big plate of broccoli could better your odds of beating breast cancer and slash your chance of getting it in the first place. It and other cruciferous vegetables boast cancer-fighting compounds that may block cancer from developing as well as keep it from spreading.

Broccoli, cabbage, watercress, kale, cauliflower, and other crucifers are rich in plant compounds called glucosinolates. The bacteria in your gut break them down into other substances — sulforaphane, indole-3-carbinol, and isothiocyanates to name a few. These, in turn, trigger cancer cells to commit suicide, a process known as apoptosis. They also help prevent cancerous changes in your cells and change the way your body uses estrogen, so less of the hormone fuels cancer growth.

Sulforaphane. This antioxidant revs up an enzyme in your body that gets rid of dangerous toxins, and eating cruciferous vegetables rich in it has been linked to a lower cancer risk. In the lab, sulforaphane slowed the growth of breast cancer cells. Experts hope it could one day prevent estrogen-positive breast cancer.

Finely shredding brassicas can take away up to 75 percent of their anti-cancer compounds in just six hours. Boiling them leaches many of these valuable compounds into the cooking water. Your best bet is to steam, microwave, or stir-fry.

DIM. In your gut, indole-3-carbinol breaks down further into Diindolylmethane (DIM). This potent compound squashes two proteins that help breast and ovarian cancer spread through your body. In fact, treating cancer cells with DIM reduced their spread an amazing 80 percent.

Experts say this may make current cancer treatments like radiation and chemotherapy more effective, since DIM could stop the cancer from spreading or at least slow it down. The compound also helps boost immune function, which may thwart cancer from ever developing.

Isothiocyanates. New research connects crucifers high in ITCs, particularly raw white turnips and Chinese cabbage, to a lower risk of breast cancer in postmenopausal women. Younger women benefited, too, but for a different reason. Premenopausal women with certain types of genes faced a much higher risk of breast cancer than other women. However, if they ate cruciferous vegetables their risk dropped significantly.

Women who eat a lot of meat should take special care to pile on the vegetables. Grilling, pan-frying, smoking, barbecuing, and even broiling meat creates PAHs and HCAs, two carcinogens linked to breast cancer. The more grilled, barbecued, or smoked meats women ate in one study, the more likely they were to develop breast cancer. If they ate lots of meat but few fruits and vegetables, their risk jumped even higher.

Loading your plate with sides of fruits and vegetables, particularly those rich in ITCs like crucifers, may offset some of that risk if you're a meat-lover. White turnips are one great source. Raw, they pack an incredible 17 times more ITCs than bok choy, another crucifer. Watercress follows close behind, with 16 times more ITCs than bok choy.

Brassicas K.O. colon cancer

Eat your brussels sprouts. You heard it a hundred times growing up, but even mom may not have known how right she was. The brussels sprouts, broccoli, cabbage, and cauliflower in the produce aisle can all protect you from colon cancer. They contain a natural plant compound called glucobrassicin, which breaks down in your belly into indole-3-carbinol (I3C). This hard-to-pronounce substance gets digested even further, eventually turning into Diindolylmethane (DIM). New evidence suggests DIM is behind the cancer-protection afforded by brassicas.

Tumors develop for two reasons. Damaged cells:

■ multiply uncontrollably, forming tumors.

■ stop responding to signals your body sends them, telling them to die.

Certain compounds, such as DIM, help damaged cells to die when they should, so they don't keep multiplying and turn cancerous. That's why experts now think that eating brassicas like broccoli and brussels sprouts may prevent colon cancer from developing and even slow the growth of existing cancer. That, in turn, could make traditional treatments more effective. Best of all, DIM does this without causing side effects, unlike medications.

How you eat them matters, though. The amount of protection you get from food depends partly on how you prepare it.

- Crucifers can lose 30 to 60 percent of their cancer-fighting compounds during cooking, but different methods yield different results. One study found cooking red cabbage over low heat on the stove or mid-range power in the microwave actually increased its cancer-fighting power.

- Raw may be the way to go. Rats that ate raw, fresh watercress, green cabbage, and broccoli for nearly four months had fewer colon cancer markers than rats on regular diets.

- Juicing doesn't work. Vegetable juice had no effect on cancer in an animal study, nor did supplements made from the protective compounds in the vegetables.

Nutritious fad: colorful cauliflower

Cauliflower comes in technicolor now. No longer boring and white, you can buy it in vivid purple, orange, and green. These color variations occasionally sprout up naturally, but growers have begun selectively breeding cauliflower to produce the colors consistently.

Why all the fuss? Colored cauliflowers contain more of certain nutrients than their white counterparts. Purple cauliflower is packed with anthocyanin, the same phytochemical found in red grapes and red wine. Orange cauliflower boasts loads of beta carotene, about 25 times more than white, while green heads have a little more vitamin C and A.

Common cabbage keeps arthritis at bay

One humble vegetable has surprising healing properties that combat infectious skin problems, strengthen weak bones, and lessen arthritis pain. The lowly cabbage, once a "poor man's" food, is finally starting to gain some respect.

Takes the ache from arthritis. Cabbage and other cruciferous vegetables boast two nutrients that improve osteoarthritis pain and keep the disease from getting worse.

■ Vitamin C reacts with iron to build healthy joint cartilage. Research suggests antioxidants like vitamin C also keep you from losing cartilage and slow the progression of osteoarthritis (OA). People who got lots of vitamin C in one study were less likely to have knee pain or see their OA worsen, while those in another study had fewer and smaller bone marrow lesions — markers of arthritis, joint pain, and worsening OA.

■ Cabbage and its fellow crucifers are also chock-full of vitamin K, which regulates the growth of bone and cartilage. Seniors with higher blood levels of vitamin K had fewer signs of hand and knee osteoarthritis in one study. Researchers think too little K may lead to shrinking cartilage and the growth of bone spurs common in arthritis.

Strengthens bones. Besides building cartilage, vitamin C may directly affect your bone health. It's a key part of the proteins that form collagen, one of the building blocks of bone, ligaments, tendons, and teeth. Plus, it stimulates your body to make osteoblasts, or bone cells. In postmenopausal women, higher vitamin C is associated with greater bone mineral density, a marker of bone strength.

Vitamin K is essential in building osteocalcin, another major protein in bones. A shortage of K weakens your bones, and studies link low-K diets to lower BMD and higher risk of bone fracture. On the other hand, boosting your vitamin K keeps you from losing calcium through urine, reduces the amount of bone your body breaks down, and increases the amount of bone in your body. In a 10-year study, women who got the least vitamin K in their diets were 30 percent more likely to fracture their hip, while other research found that men and women who got the most vitamin K were 65 percent less likely to fracture a hip.

Heals skin conditions. As early as the 1930s, scientists realized vitamin C helped heal cold sores and other lesions caused by the Herpes simplex virus. Further research showed it could help heal outbreaks twice as fast as simple waiting, probably because it enhances your immune system and fights viruses.

When it comes to vitamin K, ordinary boiled cabbage is tops. Just half a cup of cooked cabbage meets 100 percent of your daily K needs, not to mention almost half your vitamin C requirements, in only 17 calories. If you're keen to get the most vitamin C, though, start adding raw red cabbage to salads and cole slaws. A cup of chopped cabbage provides 85 percent of the day's vitamin C and about 40 percent of your vitamin K, all in a mere 28 calories.

Boost your immune system with broccoli

Two powerful cruciferous chemicals found in broccoli can rev up your rundown immune system, fending off viruses and keeping you healthier throughout the year.

DIM the lights on viruses. When you sit down to a meal with broccoli, cabbage, or kale, you're girding your immune system to fight off infections. Diindolylmethane (DIM), one of the compounds formed when you digest these foods, pumps up your immune system. Mice fed DIM had:

■ more cytokines, proteins that help regulate immune cells.

■ more active macrophages, immune cells that help kill bacteria and tumor cells.

■ twice the number of white blood cells, which fight off infection by surrounding or killing the bugs attacking your body.

What's more, mice on the DIM diet cleared invading viruses out of their bodies faster than regular mice, so they recovered from being sick quicker.

Strengthen with sulforaphane. This cruciferous compound boosts the immune system, too. In mice, it spurred on natural killer immune cells, helped produce more cytokines and lymphocytes, and stimulated other parts of the immune system. What's more, certain crucifers such as broccoli are excellent sources of vitamin C, another virus-busting nutrient. So instead of turning to supplements to fend off sickness, try a side of broccoli or brussels sprouts with your meals.

Pile on the veggies for prostate health

Serving up a side of cauliflower at least once a week can protect you from deadly forms of prostate cancer, according to exciting new findings published in the *Journal of the National Cancer Institute*. Crucifers are chock-full of natural cancer-fighting compounds, including isothiocyanates, indoles, and sulforaphane, which help protect the genetic material in your cells from damage. What's more, broccoli is particularly high in phenols, plant substances that boost your immune system and squash dangerous compounds that can lead to cancerous changes in your body. Here's what crucifers can do for your prostate.

Evade aggressive cancers. Researchers followed 29,000 men for four years. Men who ate either broccoli or cauliflower more than once a week faced half the risk of advanced, aggressive prostate cancer as men who ate the veggies less than once a month. You need all the extra protection you can get. While most prostate cancers are slow-growing and highly treatable, aggressive prostate cancer is often deadly.

Shrink prostate tumors. When rats with regular prostate cancer were fed broccoli as part of their meals, their tumors shrank a whopping 42 percent. Eating tomatoes and broccoli together had an even greater impact, shrinking tumors 52 percent. Researchers think the natural cancer-fighters in these foods slowed down the growth of prostate tumors and killed off existing tumor cells.

To see similar benefits, you need to eat about one-and-a-half cups of raw broccoli daily, along with two-and-a-half cups of fresh tomato, one cup of tomato sauce, or half a cup of tomato paste. "I think it's very doable for a man to eat a cup and a half of broccoli per day or to put broccoli on a pizza with half a cup of tomato paste," says the study's co-author Kirstie Canene-Adams. "Older men with slow-growing prostate cancer who have chosen watchful waiting over chemotherapy and radiation should seriously consider altering their diets to include more tomatoes and broccoli." You can boost your food's anti-cancer powers even more with a few tips.

- Sprinkle some curry on your cauliflower. An animal study found that a combination of PEITC, a compound in cruciferous vegetables, and curcumin, a compound in curry seasoning, stopped new prostate tumors from developing and put the breaks on existing ones. An ounce of watercress may pack enough PEITC to fight the growth of prostate cancer.

- Chew or chop your veggies. PEITC and other isothiocyanates form when the plant's cells get crushed up, for instance during chewing or chopping the vegetables. So be sure to munch your broccoli, cabbage, cauliflower, watercress, and other crucifers thoroughly to get the most prostate protection.

Curry powder

Golden spice keeps your brain sharp

Those pesky free radicals — they can make you age in so many ways. From memory loss to arthritis and even digestive problems, free radicals from metabolism and other body processes are damaging your cells all the time. But an inexpensive seasoning from your spice rack has antioxidant powers to help prevent free radical damage. That seasoning is curry powder, a spice mixture that contains lots of turmeric.

Maintain a young brain. Researchers noticed that India — where curry is king — has a rate of Alzheimer's disease that is one-quarter that of the United States. They wondered if the region's food might explain the difference.

Curry powder gets its yellow color from curcumin, a compound found in turmeric. Studies have shown curcumin blocks certain proteins that can lead to inflammation in your brain, thus fending off Alzheimer's disease. Curcumin can stop the formation of brain plaques common in Alzheimer's disease and even weaken plaques that have already built up. It also beefs up immune cells that run throughout your body gobbling up waste — including the protein plaques that build up in a brain with Alzheimer's.

This idea is more than just a theory. A study at the National University of Singapore found that people who eat curry more often tend to score better on memory tests. You can benefit by using a teaspoon or two of curry in your cooking whenever possible.

Evade inflammatory woes. The anti-inflammatory and antioxidant powers of turmeric can help you in other ways. It stops the pain and swelling of rheumatoid arthritis by blocking joint inflammation. Turmeric's active ingredient works so well that some experts even compare it to nonsteroidal anti-inflammatory drugs, which include aspirin and ibuprofen.

Curcumin may also treat digestive problems caused by inflammation run amok, like Crohn's disease or ulcerative colitis. Researchers think the spice could do some good, but they're still working to prove the idea.

Turmeric, the source of curcumin, is not for everyone. It can behave like a blood thinner, lead to kidney stones, or cause stomach upset. You shouldn't take it at all if you have gallstones or you're on a blood thinner, like warfarin or heparin. Talk to your doctor.

Savor a spicy cancer fighter

Wouldn't it be great if there were a single food you could eat to fight cancers all over your body? Try a pinch of curry. Curcumin, an active part of turmeric in curry, fights at least four types of cancer.

- Prostate cancer cells commit suicide — called apoptosis — when curcumin is around. One lab study found a mixture of curcumin and a cancer-fighter in your body nicknamed TRAIL killed about 80 percent of cancer cells. Experts think curcumin works by turning off the gene that causes prostate tumors to form.

- The extract also causes cancer-cell suicide in melanoma, one of the most deadly types of skin cancer.

- Curcumin blocks a digestive hormone that causes tumors to grow in your colon. This hormone, called neurotensin, also allows colon cancer to spread to other parts of your body.

"About a third of all colorectal cancer cells have the receptor for neurotensin," says Professor B. Mark Evers, one of the researchers who is investigating curcumin and colon cancer at the University of Texas Medical Branch at Galveston. "Thus, the concept would be sort of like what we do for breast and prostate cancer, where the main therapy involves blocking hormones. We hope to do similar things with gastrointestinal cancers that respond to this hormone."

- Doctors sometimes prescribe drugs like the pain reliever celecoxib (Celebrex) to prevent pancreatic cancer. They have found that taking curcumin along with a COX-2 drug helps it work better against cancer cells. That means you may be able to take a lower dose of the drug, possibly avoiding side effects like heart or digestive damage.

Most research on curcumin and cancer has taken place in the lab rather than on people. More studies are being done to see if curcumin will turn out to be your best cancer-fighting ally yet.

Follow the yellow brick road to diabetes defense

The ingredient in curry that makes it yellow may also help you control type 2 diabetes and sidestep its side effects. Give the credit to curcumin. This spicy pigment provides three weapons in your diabetes crusade.

Household Hint

Cook up yellow yarn to dye for

You can use turmeric as a natural dye. It creates vibrant, sunshiny yellow yarn for happy knitting. Here's how to dye two skeins or two balls of wool or cotton yarn.

- Simmer 1 ounce of ground turmeric in 3 quarts of water for 30 minutes.

- While the dye bath reduces, prepare your yarn by winding it into hanks that will allow the dye to reach all threads, yet not get tangled. Do this by winding the yarn between your hand and elbow into long loops.

- Wet the yarn and squeeze out excess water to let the dye work evenly.

- Submerge the yarn into your simmering pot and leave it for 30 minutes.

- Remove the yarn from the dye bath, and wash it with soap and water to remove excess dye. Let it hang to dry.

Battles high blood sugar. Watching what you eat is key to keeping your blood sugar in check. Do a good job, and you may be able to avoid the damaging side effects of diabetes. Lab tests found that diabetic mice who took curcumin had fewer episodes of high blood sugar and even put on less belly fat. Experts think curcumin changes the way your cells function so blood sugar doesn't get too high.

Maintains sharp eyesight. If you've had diabetes for a while, your vision may be at risk. That's because repeated episodes of high blood sugar can lead to retinopathy, or blindness caused by damage to the small blood vessels in your eyes. Poor sugar control may also bring on cataracts, a cloudiness of the lens in the front of your eye. Curcumin can help you avoid both of these vision problems caused in part by dangerous free radicals. It hunts down these unstable molecules and gobbles them up, which helps prevent the cell damage that can lead to vision problems.

Banishes nerve pain. Diabetic neuropathy — nerve damage from high blood sugar — can cause pain and tingling. You may feel it in your hands, feet, legs — really any part of your body. It's hard to treat, but curcumin may help. Lab tests show its antioxidant powers may reduce pain by calming the nerve endings.

Yam Fries with Curry

Ingredients

4 cups yams, cut into thin strips
  similar to traditional french fries

2 Tbsp olive oil

1/2 tsp salt

1 tsp white pepper

1 tsp curry powder

1/2 tsp cayenne pepper

Instructions

1. Combine olive oil and all the seasonings in a bowl and mix well.

2. Dip yam strips into oil and seasoning mixture. Coat well.

3. Spread strips on an ungreased baking sheet. Bake at 375 degrees for 20 minutes or until a fork can easily pierce the yam strips.

4. Serve warm with a dipping sauce or mustard.

(Serves 6)

Nutrition Summary by Serving

160.6 Calories (42.8 calories from fat, 26.64 percent of total); 4.8 g Fats;
1.6 g Protein; 28.4 g Carbohydrates; 0.0 mg Cholesterol; 4.4 g Fiber; 205.8 mg Sodium

Protect your heart with curry power

People have used turmeric as a medicine for centuries, but experts are still finding new ways it may help you. Now researchers are looking into how it can keep your heart healthy.

Trims down your heart. Curcumin, the yellow part of turmeric, may protect you from an enlarged heart. That can happen if you have high blood pressure. And while having a big heart may sound like a good thing, it's not good for you.

"Whether you are young or old, male or female, the larger your heart is, the higher your risk is for developing heart attacks or heart failure in the future," says Dr. Peter Liu, a cardiologist in the Peter Munk Cardiac Center at the Canadian Institutes of Health Research.

Lab studies show curcumin blocks certain enzymes in your body that can lead to heart enlargement. If you already have an enlarged heart, curcumin may prevent the damage from progressing to heart failure.

Guards your vessels. Curcumin may also prevent heart disease and fight high cholesterol. It does this by strengthening blood vessel walls, keeping blood cells from clumping together, and stopping extra LDL cholesterol — the "bad" kind — from forming. Experts think curcumin may work even better than some other powerful plant protectors, like quercetin from apples and onions.

Dairy

Delicious way to dodge diabetes

Diabetes may be easier to avoid than you think. Nine out of 10 cases of type 2 diabetes can be attributed to our choices and habits, studies say. That means the power to avoid diabetes is in your hands right now. Why not start by eating low-fat dairy products every day? These foods may look ordinary, but researchers say they've already shown their mettle against diabetes.

Harness the power of protein. In a 10-year study of over 37,000 women, those who ate the most low-fat dairy products were 20 percent less likely to be diagnosed with diabetes than those who ate the least. The Harvard researchers behind the study think milk proteins may help prevent high blood sugar.

Remember, insulin is in charge of keeping your blood sugar down, so type 2 diabetes occurs when your body has trouble making insulin or your cells have trouble using it. Fortunately, the milk proteins in yogurt, milk, and other dairy foods are "insulinotropic." That means they encourage your body to make and use more insulin. But not all dairy products can do this. The saturated fat in high-fat dairy products may wipe out the positive effects of milk proteins, so stick with low-fat dairy products.

Fight back with calcium and vitamin D. Yet milk proteins aren't the only anti-diabetes weapon in your dairy arsenal. According to a Tufts University study, people who take in three to five servings of dairy a day are 15 percent less likely to get type 2 diabetes than people who only get one-and-a-half servings. But Tufts researchers think calcium and vitamin D are the nutrients that battle diabetes. For example, they point out that calcium is a key ingredient in the insulin-producing process, so they suspect that shortage of calcium or vitamin D may interfere with your body's ability to make insulin. What's more, some studies show that shortfalls in vitamin D and calcium may make it tougher for your body to use insulin to control your blood sugar. So getting enough of these nutrients may help you retain control over your blood sugar the same way milk proteins would.

These studies aren't the final word on diabetes prevention, but they do come from two of America's leading hubs of nutritional research. So try replacing some of your favorite fatty foods with chilled skim milk, a creamy serving of nonfat yogurt, or a slice of low-fat cheese. Just a few servings of low-fat dairy each day may help you dodge diabetes for life.

Yak cheese: a heart-smart choice

You love cheese but you know all that saturated fat can't be good for your heart. Soon you may have another alternative to cheese from cows — yak cheese from Tibet. Yaks are long-haired cattle found in the Himalayan mountains. The cheese made from their milk may be healthier for you in three ways.

- It has higher levels of heart-healthy polyunsaturated fat than cheese from cows.

- It has three times more omega-3 fatty acids and four times as much conjugated linoleic acid — two fats that may help fight heart disease.

- It has less total fat as well as less saturated fat than regular cheese.

Yak cheese tastes like a medium cheddar, but it's pricey and only available from gourmet food stores and Internet vendors. But a cheese this promising probably won't stay pricey and rare for long, so keep checking for it at your local stores.

Burn fat faster with a creamy treat

The smooth, silky texture of yogurt may make you think of dessert, but choose wisely and it could help you burn off body fat instead.

According to a Purdue University study, young women who averaged 1,242 mg of daily calcium from eating dairy foods reduced their body fat over an 18-month period, but those who got less dairy calcium accumulated more fat. Earlier research from the University of Tennessee found similar results. Those who ate three 6-ounce servings of yogurt lost 81 percent more body fat in the stomach area than people who ate less yogurt. That's good news because fat around your stomach may raise your risk of heart disease, diabetes, and stroke more than fat found elsewhere.

Yogurt's fat-fighting secret may be its calcium. When you don't get enough calcium, your body may take that as a sign that you're starving. To "rescue" you, it pumps out more of a calcium-related hormone that makes your body store extra fat. But when you get enough calcium, those hormone levels drop, and your body is free to burn fat away. Other compounds in dairy may also pitch in to help trim the fat, which is why eating dairy is better than taking a calcium supplement.

If you want to try this, you can get up to 1,245 mg of calcium by eating three containers of low-fat yogurt daily or drinking four cups of nonfat milk. Just be sure to use yogurt or milk as a replacement for other fatty foods in your diet, and stick with the low-fat or nonfat versions. Otherwise, the added fat and calories may lead to weight gain.

Say cheese for a cavity-free smile

Dairy foods like cheese, yogurt, and milk are a triple threat against cavities. Here's how they can help you avoid the dentist's drill.

- Dairy foods are high in calcium and phosphorous. These mighty minerals help strengthen the bone around your teeth and fortify your tooth enamel against cavities.

- When the bacteria on your teeth turn sugar into acids, those acids can eat away at your teeth and cause cavities. But cheese can raise the pH values in your mouth, making it less acidic. Just a bite or two of cheddar, Monterey Jack, or mozzarella after a meal or snack may make all the difference.

- Cheese may help increase the amount of saliva in your mouth, which helps wash away harmful acids on your teeth.

Uncover the truth about milk and bones

You may have heard news stories saying calcium can't prevent disabling fractures from osteoporosis, but don't give up milk, cheese, and yogurt yet. Find out the hidden truths behind the headlines, and see why women aren't the only ones who can still use calcium to save their bones.

Evaluate study stats. At first, the large Women's Health Initiative study reported that women who get more calcium are just as likely to experience a fracture as women who get little. But then researchers discovered how many study participants had not been taking their calcium supplements regularly. Among women who did take the supplements regularly, calcium lowered the risk of hip fracture by 29 percent — nearly one third.

On top of that, a new study of both men and women found that those who got 1,200 mg of calcium daily were 72 percent less likely to experience a fracture. But the researchers warn that fracture risk only dropped while study participants were getting the full amount of calcium. The protection vanished quickly once they stopped.

This probably happened because your body "robs Peter to pay Paul." When you do not take in enough calcium, it's pulled from your bones to maintain normal nerve and muscle functions. That makes your bones weaker and more likely to break. Calcium supplements can help, but some experts say you get more and better nutrition if you get calcium from foods. Plus, some studies suggest that calcium isn't the only nutrient in dairy foods that can strengthen your bones. Nutrients like vitamin D and the whey protein found in some dairy products may also help.

Recognize who is at risk. Many people don't realize that nearly one out of five people who get osteoporosis are men — and they're even more likely than women to die after a bone fracture. But now research from Australia's Deakin University suggests that dairy foods may help fight off these dangers. The Australian scientists found that older men who drank two glasses of specially fortified low-fat milk daily lost 1.6 percent less bone than men who didn't. That may not sound like much, but scientists say it can make a significant difference in your risk of a disabling fracture over the long haul. The specially fortified milk also lowered levels of a hormone that contributes to bone loss.

The milk used in the study provided 1,000 mg of calcium and 800 IU of vitamin D in just two glasses. You won't find that much in the milk you buy in stores. But you can still get the same amount of calcium by drinking two 8-ounce glasses of skim milk and eating a container of yogurt. To equal the amount of vitamin D as those in the study, drink a couple of glasses of milk, enjoy fatty fish, and eat foods fortified with vitamin D to start. Then talk to your doctor about other ways to get the right amount of this critical vitamin.

Key to building better bones

Good news for women who don't like taking pills. Calcium from foods may be safer for your heart and remarkably better for your bones.

Women who take calcium supplements are more likely to have heart attacks than women who don't, suggests a new study from the University of Auckland. On top of that, a study from Washington University in St. Louis discovered that women who got 830 mg of calcium from foods had a higher bone mass density than women who took 1,000 mg of supplements. The researchers point out that your body can only absorb 35 percent of the calcium in supplements but can get much more of the calcium in foods. What's more, they think calcium-loaded foods may cause your body to make more of the kind of estrogen that strengthens bones.

Dairy: the answer to colon cancer

Promising news about colon cancer and dairy has come out of the Land of the Midnight Sun. Researchers from Sweden's Karolinska

Institute followed more than 45,000 men for six years, keeping track of what they ate and whether they got colon cancer. They discovered that men who ate more servings of dairy foods were the ones least likely to get colon cancer. In fact, men who drank at least 1 1/2 glasses of milk each day slashed their risk by one-third compared to men who drank two or fewer per week. The study also found that the more dietary calcium the men got, the more their colon cancer risk dropped. Calcium may help prevent colon cancer for several reasons.

■ It binds bile acids and ionized fatty acids. This keeps them from irritating your colon lining in ways that may cause cancer.

■ Cell overgrowth has also been linked to cancer, but calcium may regulate cell responses and signaling to keep the cells of your colon lining from multiplying out of control.

■ Calcium may help prevent cancer-causing agents from attacking the lining of the colon.

But that's not the end of the story. The Swedish researchers say calcium alone wasn't enough to explain all the cancer-fighting power milk showed in their study. Animal studies suggest that the milk proteins, conjugated linoleic acid, and compounds called sphingolipids in milk may also help stop cancer before it starts. Milk's vitamin D and magnesium may help prevent colon cancer as well. So try a glass or two of milk a day. You might end up with a whole team of nutrients to keep colon cancer away from you.

Eggs

Fit eggs into a heart-smart diet

Like Dr. Richard Kimble in *The Fugitive*, eggs may have been framed for a crime they didn't commit. Eggs and their cholesterol have long been blamed for heart attacks, strokes, and high cholesterol, but now experts have discovered three good reasons why eggs can be part of a heart-healthy diet.

Egg myths unscrambled. Eggs got their bad reputation back when experts thought an egg's 200 milligrams (mg) of cholesterol automatically turned into 200 mg of blood cholesterol. But a study out of Michigan State University found that people who ate four or more eggs a week had lower cholesterol levels than people who ate one egg or less. How is that possible? Doctors now know that little of your cholesterol is brought in by foods. Instead, most of it is made by your liver. But be aware that the real villains — the saturated fats and trans fats in foods — cause your liver to produce even more cholesterol than usual. That's probably why the American Heart Association (AHA) recommends limiting saturated fats to only 7 percent of the calories in your diet — approximately 16 grams of saturated fat if you eat 2,000 calories a day.

> For more information on the nutritional benefits of eggs, see *Fight vision loss and win* in the Lutein & zeaxanthin chapter.

The AHA also recommends limiting cholesterol to 300 mg a day if you're a healthy adult or to 200 mg if you have heart disease, high cholesterol, or diabetes. This means you can enjoy approximately one egg per day if you limit or eliminate saturated fats, trans fats, and cholesterol from other foods.

Surprising truth about LDL. Studies have suggested that one-third of all people are extra sensitive to food cholesterol — meaning the food they eat causes a higher-than-normal rise in blood cholesterol levels. These people are called "hyper-responders."

A University of Connecticut study found that hyper-responders who ate three eggs a day for 30 days developed higher LDL and HDL cholesterol levels, but that extra LDL may have more bark than bite. Recent research reveals that larger LDL cholesterol particles are less likely to endanger your heart while small, dense particles are a sign of heart disease risk. The LDL added when hyper-responders ate eggs was made up entirely of the safer large particles.

Guide to healthy eating. A famous Harvard study of more than 37,000 men and 80,000 women found that people who ate up to one egg a day were no more likely to experience heart disease, stroke, or death from heart disease than those who rarely ate eggs. Only people with diabetes were more likely to develop heart disease from eating an egg a day.

In spite of the positive findings for eggs, some studies have still suggested eggs may raise cholesterol — so don't go hog wild. Instead, use these guidelines for heart healthy eating.

- Use egg substitutes or avoid eggs on days when you expect to eat high-cholesterol, high-saturated-fat dishes such as meats.

- Enjoy one egg on days when you expect to eat little or no cholesterol or saturated fat.

Coming soon: the hypoallergenic egg

Imagine eating an egg safely even though you're normally allergic to them. German and Swiss chemists say they've developed a process that makes eggs 100 times less allergenic than a regular raw egg, but without changing the egg's taste or texture. So someday soon, you might not only be able to eat eggs, but perhaps even mayonnaise, desserts, and more. Stay tuned for more on this egg-citing development.

Household Hint

Get egg-cellent results in your garden

The same egg you eat for breakfast can
also be a problem-solver for your plants.
Here's how.

- Slugs don't like walking on eggshells
  any more than you do. Save your eggshells and crush
  them. Then spread the pieces around any plant you
  want to protect. Surround the plant completely for a
  slug-proof zone.

- Crushed eggshells are also a great source of calcium —
  which is just what you need to prevent blossom end
  rot on your tomato plants. You can also sprinkle them
  into the soil of your houseplants.

- Another way to get eggshell calcium to houseplants is
  to save the water you use to boil eggs. Once it cools,
  water your plants with it and see how much better
  they grow.

Breakfast trick melts pounds and inches

Diet plans that leave you hungry are a terrible idea. Either you're too
starved to think straight or you feel guilty because you broke down
and had a snack when you weren't supposed to. But one small change
can help you feel full, eat less, and kiss those extra pounds good-bye.

According to a study from St. Louis University, overweight women
who ate an egg breakfast took in fewer lunchtime calories and
carbohydrates at lunch than women who ate a bagel-based breakfast.
But that's just the beginning. Over the next day and a half, egg eaters

also totaled fewer calories, fewer grams of protein, and fewer carbohydrates than bagel-eaters. Even though both breakfasts had the same number of calories, egg-eating women took longer to become hungry again. This happened because an egg simply "sticks to your ribs" better than a bagel with cream cheese. As a result, you don't get hungry quickly and you're not so tempted to shovel in extra calories.

A similar study funded by the National Egg Board suggests this tactic can work even better if you stick with it. This time people who participated in the study ate the bagel breakfast or egg breakfast five days a week for two months. They also ate a reduced-calorie diet. But in the end, the egg eaters still lost more pounds and reported higher energy levels than bagel eaters. They also lowered their waist measurements by up to 83 percent more.

So if you've had trouble losing weight or sticking with your diet, why not try an egg for breakfast? Enjoy it scrambled, boiled, or poached just like the people in the studies. But don't accompany your egg with bacon, sausage, or other fatty foods. Instead, try it with a couple of slices of toast and low-calorie jam or jelly. You may be delighted to discover how much easier weight loss can be — and how much better you look and feel.

Fish

Help yourself to heart-healthy fish

Your heart works hard to keep you alive. The least you could do is reward it for its efforts. That's where fish comes in. Adding fish to your diet just might add years to your life. Population studies show a link between fish consumption and fewer deaths from heart disease. You don't have to go overboard, either. Just one or two fish dishes a week can slash your risk of dying from heart disease by 50 percent. Fish also reduces your risk of sudden cardiac death.

The key to fish's success lies with its omega-3 fatty acids, docosahexaenoic acid (DHA) and eicosapentaenoic acid (EPA). These essential fatty acids help your heart in a variety of ways, such as:

- reducing platelet clumping, a factor in blood clots that can trigger heart attacks or strokes.

- lowering triglycerides, dangerous fats in your blood that increase your risk of heart disease. Omega-3 can slash triglyceride levels by at least 30 percent in people with high or normal triglyceride levels.

- helping to prevent arrhythmia, or irregular heartbeat, and lowering your blood pressure. Just 3 grams of EPA and DHA lead to a drop of 5 millimeters of mercury (mm Hg) in systolic blood pressure and 3 mm Hg drop in diastolic blood pressure.

- increasing LDL particle size, making them less likely to oxidize and become dangerous.

- stunting the growth of plaque in your arteries, protecting against free radical damage, and enhancing the actions of insulin.

More evidence for the importance of omega-3 comes from a recent study that found DHA levels were lower in people who experience cardiovascular events, like heart attack or stroke. On the other hand, a Japanese study found a 19 percent reduction in coronary events in people who took EPA. Of course, the Japanese also eat more fish than most people.

Eating more fish is not a bad idea. Sticking to a Mediterranean diet, which includes a high fish intake, can help lower mortality, according to one study. A diet that includes more fish and plant food and less red and processed meat means a lower risk of deep vein thrombosis, a dangerous condition that includes painful blood clots in your legs or clots that block the flow of blood to your lungs.

Enjoy fish two to three times a week as part of a healthy diet. Your heart will thank you — without skipping a beat.

Powerful weapon protects against stroke

A stroke can drastically change — or end — your life within seconds. But if you take the time to eat more fish, you can gain 'round-the-clock protection.

There are two main types of stroke. An ischemic stroke happens when a blockage in an artery cuts off blood and oxygen to the brain. During a hemorrhagic stroke, a blood vessel bursts, leading to bleeding in the brain. One study suggests that eating fish just one to three times a month can protect you from ischemic stroke. Another study, which tracked more than 4,000 older men and women for 12 years, found that those who ate tuna or baked or broiled fish up to four times a week had a 27 percent lower risk of stroke than those who ate fish less than once a month. But don't go overboard. Some experts say that eating too much fish — like five or six servings per week — may boost your risk for hemorrhagic stroke.

Fish may help prevent strokes for several reasons. High blood pressure ranks as the No. 1 risk factor for stroke, and the omega-3 fatty acids in fish help lower your blood pressure. They also have anti-inflammatory and anti-clotting powers, which makes them powerful weapons against stroke.

According to a German study, low blood levels of vitamin B12 mean an increased risk for stroke. One way to boost your B12 intake is to eat more fish. Good sources include oysters, clams, crabs, salmon, sardines, trout, herring, pollock, flounder, sole, lobster, tuna, halibut, and swordfish.

To lower your risk of stroke, eat a diet low in sodium and high in potassium. Along with fish, it should include plenty of fruits, vegetables, whole grains, and cereal fiber.

Safe ways to enjoy seafood

Perhaps you've stopped eating fish because you're worried about mercury poisoning or pollutants, such as chemicals called polychlorinated biphenyls (PCBs). Recent studies may relieve those worries somewhat. It turns out that cooking the fish and removing the skin reduces contaminants by an average of 35 percent in salmon and 50 percent in Great Lakes fish such as trout, bass, and bluefish. Researchers tested baking, boiling, microwaving, and pan frying, and all produced a substantial loss in pollutants, which they think dripped out with the melted fat. Other research found that simply removing the belly and back fat from fish can slash PCB content up to 40 percent.

If you're worried about getting too much mercury, check out the handy calculator at *www.gotmercury.org*. Just plug in your weight plus the type and amount of fish you eat in a week to see if you're in the safe range. Choose canned light tuna rather than canned albacore tuna. Other low-mercury options include clams, flounder, halibut, pollock, fresh or frozen salmon, shrimp, and tilapia.

Fight diabetes with a fishy food plan

Having diabetes means having to make some dietary changes. One of the smartest changes you can make is to add more fish to your diet. Loaded with omega-3 fatty acids, fish can help you manage your diabetes. This disease is uncommon in Greenland and among Alaskan Eskimos, populations known for eating lots of fish. In a study of older Dutch people, those who ate more fish were less likely to develop diabetes or glucose intolerance.

Omega-3 fatty acids can lower triglycerides by 20 to 50 percent in healthy people — and even more for people with high triglycerides, including those with diabetes. It may improve insulin sensitivity and glucose metabolism and even help you sidestep serious nerve, kidney, and eye complications.

The American Diabetes Association recommends eating at least two servings of fish per week, mostly because of omega-3's ability to lower triglyceride levels in people with type 2 diabetes. Omega-3 from fish also helps reduce heart attacks and strokes. As an added bonus, fish often takes the place of foods high in harmful saturated fat, like red meat.

Eating more fish and less red meat was one strategy of the Mediterranean Lifestyle Program, a diabetes treatment approach involving several dietary and lifestyle changes. One or two years of following this program proved more successful than usual diabetes care.

Make room for fish in your diabetes management plan, and you'll reel in plenty of benefits.

Easy way to boost your brainpower

Maybe you forget what you were about to say, misplace your car keys, or occasionally joke about having a "senior moment." But, contrary to popular belief, a slowing brain and memory loss are not a natural part of growing older. If you are afraid of losing your memories, try adding some fish to your plate today. It can keep your brain and memory sharp.

Reap the benefits of fish oil. In one study of more than 800 people aged 65 to 94, those who ate fish once a week or more had a 60 percent less risk of developing Alzheimer's disease compared to those who rarely or never ate fish. Another study involving people with an average age of 76 measured the levels of docosahexaenoic acid (DHA), a type of omega-3 fatty acid found in fatty fish. Researchers found that people with the highest blood levels of DHA were nearly 40 percent less likely to develop Alzheimer's and 47 percent less likely to have dementia of any kind.

Here's why fish may help. Alzheimer's disease has been linked to inflammatory factors in the brain, and fish oil — both eicosapentaenoic acid (EPA) and DHA — reduces inflammation. People with Alzheimer's also have lower levels of DHA in their brain, so eating more fish can help correct that. Plus, DHA may block the buildup of brain proteins associated with Alzheimer's.

Several studies show that fish protects you from all forms of dementia — not just the dreaded Alzheimer's. Eating fish can help slow mental decline and improve performance on mental tests. The key is to adjust your diet so you take in more omega-3 and less omega-6. Too much of the latter can promote inflammation.

Rev up your vitamin B12. Fish also gives you vitamin B12, which helps you avoid a common vitamin deficiency among older adults that affects your nerves and other vital systems. You may have trouble thinking or walking, and low vitamin B12 status can lead to more rapid mental decline.

Are you getting enough? Find out how much you need and the best foods that have it. If you're over 70, you may need much higher doses of vitamin B12. One study found that the minimum dose to correct a mild vitamin B12 deficiency is 600 micrograms per day. You can also try to get more vitamin B12 through your diet. Good seafood sources of vitamin B12 include oysters, clams, crabs, salmon, sardines, trout, herring, pollock, flounder, sole, lobster, tuna, halibut, and swordfish.

In some cases, food and supplements won't help. Some people, as they age, don't produce enough of a substance in the stomach called intrinsic factor, which you need to absorb vitamin B12. You may need injections instead. A simple blood test can determine if you have a vitamin B12 deficiency.

Clam up to save your memory

When it comes to a better memory, remember nutrients like selenium and iron. In a Chinese study, people with lower selenium levels had lower scores on mental tests. People were more likely to experience mental decline as their selenium levels decreased, according to a French study. And Penn State researchers found that iron status has an effect on women's mental performance.

Luckily shellfish, especially clams, contain plenty of selenium and iron. In fact, 3 ounces of clams provides 41.3 micrograms of selenium, or 59 percent of the Daily Value, and 23.77 milligrams of iron for a whopping 132 percent of the Daily Value.

Brighten your mood with seafood

It may not be a traumatic event, like the loss of a loved one, that triggers depression. Diet can also play a key role. Simple dietary habits, such as eating less fish and gobbling up more saturated fat and sugar, may contribute to depression. But you can help yourself kick that blue mood.

Eat more fish. Several studies suggest fish and the oils they contain, especially the omega-3 fatty acids docosahexaenoic acid (DHA) and eicosapentaenoic acid (EPA), protect against depression. Among populations that eat a lot of fish, rates of depression are much lower.

People with low levels of DHA also have low levels of serotonin, the brain's feel-good chemical. Most antidepressants, including Prozac, work by boosting serotonin levels — and fish does the same thing.

Get the right kind of fat. Because fat makes up about 60 percent of the human brain, the type of fat you eat makes a big difference. Most people get too much omega-6 fatty acids, the kind found in vegetable oils, and not enough omega-3, which helps fight inflammation. Depression and inflammatory diseases often go hand-in-hand. In a small Ohio State University study of 43 older people, those with higher blood ratios of omega-6 to omega-3 were at greater risk for both depression and inflammatory diseases. In a sort of vicious cycle, depressive symptoms and the omega-6 to omega-3 ratios worked together to make things worse than either alone.

Fish oil capsules have been used to treat bipolar disorder, and EPA may help treat people with schizophrenia. But even healthy people can benefit from eating more fish. A recent University of Pittsburgh study found that eating omega-3 fats may make you less impulsive and depressed and easier to get along with.

To boost your omega-3 intake, good bets include sardines, salmon, herring, and mackerel. Aim for two servings of fatty fish per week. At the same time, cut back on omega-6 fatty acids by avoiding deep-fried foods and swapping soybean and corn oil for healthier canola or olive oil.

Keep an eye on fish for better vision

Concerned about your eyesight? Look no further than fish. This tasty dish from the deep may protect your eyes from serious conditions that affect your vision.

Cut down on cataracts. Cataracts can cloud your vision, but here's some sunny news. According to a Tufts University study, eating fish three or more times per week can lower your risk of developing cataracts by 11 percent, while a high intake of omega-3 fatty acids can reduce your risk of cataract surgery by 12 percent. As usual, fish's omega-3 content gets the credit for its success. It affects the composition of the membrane in your eye's lens and also fights free radicals. That's why oily, fatty fish is best. Choose salmon, herring, tuna, or mackerel.

Fight against AMD. Fatty fish also guards your eyes against age-related macular degeneration (AMD), the leading cause of blindness in older people. When you have macular degeneration, the central part of your retina, known as the macula, breaks down. Both fish intake and omega-3 intake reduced the risk of macular degeneration in the U.S. Twin Study of Age-Related Macular Degeneration. Another small study found that eating two or more servings of fish per week could cut your risk of degenerative eye disease nearly in half.

For more information on fish oil, see the Omega-3 fatty acids chapter.

Inflammation may play a role in macular degeneration — and that's where omega-3 comes in. Omega-3 may promote healthy eye tissue and help regulate inflammatory and immune responses in the retina. A recent study of mice determined that omega-3 suppressed inflammation in the retina. It may also protect against blindness caused by abnormal blood vessel growth, such as retinopathy or certain types of macular degeneration.

Keep your eyesight sharp. You can have good vision into your 90s by eating more fish and making some simple lifestyle changes. Besides adding fish to your diet, try to quit smoking and lose weight. Both cigarettes and obesity increase your risk for these vision-stealing conditions.

Surround your joints with gentle relief

Fish oil fights inflammation, making it an ideal remedy for painful rheumatoid arthritis (RA). When you have RA, your body turns on itself. Your immune system, which normally fights off viruses and other invaders, instead attacks your joints. Studies show omega-3 supplements can have a modest effect on rheumatoid arthritis symptoms. In fact, at least 13 studies show positive effects for fish oil. Making dietary changes, like taking fish oil supplements, is a practical, easy way to take control of RA.

Keep in mind it may take a while — about two to three months — to see any effect. Experts recommend starting with a higher dose, then using a lower dose for maintenance. When you combine omega-3 with an anti-inflammation diet low in arachidonic acid, a type of omega-6 fatty acid, the results are even more pronounced. With fewer tender and swollen joints, you'll improve your quality of life.

As an added bonus, omega-3 can help you cut back on non-steroidal anti-inflammatory drugs (NSAIDs) and potentially toxic medications. A recent British study found that 39 percent of people taking cod liver oil, rich in omega-3, were able to slash their dose of NSAIDs by more than 30 percent. By swapping fish oil for drugs, you lessen your risk of dangerous side effects without sacrificing relief. Just make sure to tell your doctor about any supplements you're taking.

'Magic' pill burns fat faster

Exercise does wonders for any weight-loss program. But popping some fish oil before a workout gives you even better results, according to a recent study. Overweight people who took 6 grams of fish oil daily and either ran or walked for 45 minutes three times a week lost an average of 3.3 pounds over 12 weeks. Those who took sunflower oil had only minor weight loss. To boost the activity of fat-burning enzymes, take 2 grams of fish oil capsules two hours before your workout.

Soothe inflammatory bowel disease

Everyone gets an upset stomach or deals with occasional irregularity. But when you have Crohn's disease or ulcerative colitis, you have much more serious problems. Symptoms can include rectal pain, cramping, bloody diarrhea, nausea, loss of appetite, fever, painful stomach spasms, and unexplained weight loss. Collectively, these digestive conditions are known as inflammatory bowel disease, or IBD. While IBD requires a doctor's care and medicine, fish may provide an additional — and natural — remedy.

Crohn's disease. Researchers noticed that Eskimos, big fish eaters, rarely suffered from inflammatory bowel disease. That led them to realize the importance of fish oil. Both eicosapentaenoic acid (EPA) and docosahexaenoic acid (DHA) are considered essential fatty acids, the kind your body needs but does not produce on its own. You can only get them through your diet.

The lack of essential fatty acids could play a role in inflammatory bowel disease. In one study, more than 25 percent of people with chronic intestinal disorders, mostly Crohn's disease, lacked essential fatty acids. Fish oil supplements not only correct this shortage, they also add anti-inflammatory protection. In Crohn's disease, as with many inflammatory conditions, your body's immune system turns on itself. Because fish oil fights inflammation, it makes sense that fish could provide relief from this condition.

As expected, some studies show that fish oil supplements lead to significantly fewer relapses. The best results come from using the enterically coated free-fatty-acid form of omega-3, the type your body absorbs best. In a study using this form, 59 percent of people in the fish-oil group remained in remission after one year, compared to only 26 percent in the placebo group.

Ulcerative colitis. Fish oil also shows promise for this serious condition. Two studies showed benefits, while another showed a decrease in the need for corticosteroids. For both Crohn's disease and ulcerative colitis, the dosage makes a difference. Studies using the lowest dose of fish oil did not report any benefits.

It's too early to say for sure if fish oil can help, but it's worth asking your doctor about fish oil supplements. For a tastier solution, you can also simply eat more fish.

Smart advice for supplements

Can't stand fish? Even if you're an absolute landlubber, you can still reap the benefits of omega-3 fatty acids. Simply opt for fish oil supplements. For best results, choose salmon or tuna oil rather than cod liver oil. You get more omega-3, plus a lower risk of vitamin A toxicity. Make sure you get 1 gram combined DHA and EPA, and avoid brands that add lemon oil. Always store open bottles of supplements in the refrigerator, a trick that cuts down on fishy belches. You may need large doses to match the effects achieved in clinical studies, but every bit helps.

You can also find foods fortified with omega-3, including yogurt and orange juice. But sometimes, as with eggs, they may not be worth the extra cost.

Catch a fish and catch your breath

Breathing through gills — that's what asthma feels like sometimes. Instead of struggling to breathe like a fish out of water, try adding more fish to your diet.

Some studies suggest that eating fish helps lung function and lowers the prevalence of asthma. That's because of the omega-3 fatty acids found in fish. Asthma involves chronic inflammation of the respiratory tract, so the anti-inflammatory effects of omega-3 may help. The key is to adjust the ratio of omega-6 to omega-3 fatty acids in your diet so the pro-inflammatory omega-6 fatty acids don't overpower the omega-3 and run wild.

In a study of elite athletes who suffer from exercise-induced bronchoconstriction, taking fish oil supplements helped reduce the narrowing of their airways and their use of medication. But not all studies of omega-3 supplementation have shown improvement in asthma symptoms. More encouraging news comes from a Dutch study, which found that eating fish reduces the risk of asthma in children by 66 percent.

Fish protects your lungs from more than just asthma. It also helps guard against chronic obstructive pulmonary disease (COPD), a deadly combination of emphysema and bronchitis. One study found that a high intake of fish, along with fruits, vegetables, and whole grains, can cut the risk of COPD in half. On the other hand, those who ate lots of refined grains, cured and red meats, desserts, and French fries found themselves four times more likely to develop COPD.

Make fish a regular part of a healthy diet, and you'll breathe easier.

Fortify your body against disease

Eating fish several times a week will help you battle everything from a mild cold to the more serious conditions of multiple sclerosis (MS) and cancer.

Strengthen your immune system. Sick of sniffling, sneezing, and feeling stuffed-up? Don't rely on cold medicine. Give your immune system a boost by eating more fish. You can avoid colds with cold-water fish like salmon, mackerel, and herring. Rich in omega-3 fatty acids, these fish block inflammation, which increases airflow and guards your lungs from colds and respiratory infections. Two servings of fatty fish a week should help keep you healthy. But other types of seafood also offer protection. Shellfish, such as oysters, lobsters, crabs, and clams, contain selenium. This trace mineral helps your white blood cells produce cytokines, proteins that help fend off flu viruses.

Landlubbers can get anti-inflammatory protection from omega-3 supplements or other sources of omega-3, like flaxseed oil or walnuts.

Manage MS with fish oil. Everyone should eat more fish, but people with multiple sclerosis may have added incentive. Multiple sclerosis, a chronic inflammatory disease that affects the central nervous system, comes with symptoms that include double vision, muscle weakness, fatigue, pain, and depression.

It also features high levels of inflammation in the blood, caused by blood proteins called matrix metalloproteinase-9 (MMP-9). A recent small study found that omega-3 fatty acids, the kind found in fish, reduce MMP-9 levels by 58 percent in people with MS. Other studies have found that people with MS taking fish oil capsules see their disability progress more slowly and suffer fewer relapses. While MS has no cure, fish may provide some relief from this debilitating condition.

Serve salmon to protect your prostate. What you put on your plate may protect your prostate as well. Swedish researchers found that people who ate fatty fish, like salmon, once or more per week reduced their risk of prostate cancer by 43 percent compared to those who never ate fish. They also determined that those who ate the most marine fatty acids, compared to the least, had a reduced risk of 30 percent.

The benefit depends on variations of the COX-2 gene, which plays a key role in fatty acid metabolism and inflammation. For those with a different form of the gene, eating fatty fish like salmon once or more per week resulted in a 72 percent lower risk. Those with the more common form of the gene showed no link between fish intake and prostate cancer risk. Since you don't know which form of the COX-2 gene you have, you may want to play it safe and eat more fatty fish.

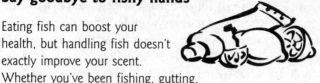
Flaxseed

Super seed saves your heart

When it comes to heart health, flaxseed gets right to the heart of the
matter. This miracle food contains nutrients that coat your arteries like
a nonstick spray, keeping your blood flowing smoothly. It lowers cholesterol, high blood pressure, and your risk of heart disease.

Clobbers cholesterol. Sweep artery-clogging cholesterol right out of
your system with this little seed. Flaxseed lowers total and LDL, or
bad, cholesterol without affecting your good HDL cholesterol levels.
Like oatmeal, flaxseed is a good source of soluble fiber, the kind that
helps lower cholesterol. Mucilage, the type of soluble fiber found in
flaxseed, works like other forms of sticky fiber. It slows down food as

it passes through your stomach and small intestines so HDL particles have more time to pick up cholesterol and whisk it to your liver, which converts it to bile and gets rid of it. Flaxseed also contains estrogen-like chemicals called lignans, which seem to have cholesterol-lowering properties. Lignans may work by affecting enzymes involved in cholesterol metabolism. Researchers found that eating two to six tablespoons of ground flax daily for as little as four weeks lowered total cholesterol by 9 percent and LDL cholesterol up to 18 percent in healthy young adults, those with moderately high cholesterol levels, and postmenopausal women.

Hammers high blood pressure. Some studies show that an increase in alpha-linolenic acid (ALA), the type of omega-3 fatty acid found in flaxseed, leads to a decrease in blood pressure. A diet rich in fiber may also lower your blood pressure. One tablespoon of ground flaxseed provides 1.8 grams of ALA and 2.2 grams of fiber, which includes both soluble and insoluble forms.

Halts heart disease. In addition to fighting high cholesterol and high blood pressure, flaxseed takes aim at other risk factors for heart disease. It fights inflammation — a key player in heart disease — by blocking pro-inflammatory eicosanoids, cytokines, and platelet activating factor. Studies also show that ALA lowers the risk of heart attacks and heart disease. It reduces blood clotting, which contributes to heart attacks and strokes, and prevents abnormal heart rhythms.

When adding high-fiber foods like flaxseed to your diet, make sure to do so gradually. Too much fiber too quickly can lead to gas, bloating, and stomach cramps. You also want to drink plenty of water.

A little flaxseed goes a long way. Just one or two tablespoons a day can give you incredible health insurance. Easy ways to add it to your diet include sprinkling roasted, ground flaxseeds on cereal, yogurt, cottage cheese, and salads. Mix flaxseed into batter for pancakes or waffles, use it for baking breads, muffins, or cookies, and add some to meatloaf, casseroles, and burgers. You can even replace fat in recipes with flaxseed. Just swap three tablespoons of ground flax for one tablespoon of shortening, butter, margarine, or oil.

Because of flaxseed's many health benefits, manufacturers are finding ways to add it to some surprising foods. Foods that contain it include energy bars, sausage, bread, yogurt, and even ice cream.

Flaxseed foils hot flashes

If the hot flashes that often accompany menopause have you hot under the collar, flaxseed may give you the chance to cool down. In a recent Mayo Clinic study, women with bothersome hot flashes took 40 grams of crushed flaxseed daily. The frequency of their hot flashes decreased 50 percent over six weeks, and the women reported improvements in mood, joint or muscle pain, chills, and sweating.

Flaxseed works because it's a phytoestrogen, or a plant-based estrogen source. Lignans in flax also have weak estrogen-like characteristics. While flax may not help everyone, it may be a safer alternative to hormone replacement therapy or drug treatments, which come with unwanted side effects.

Easy way to protect your prostate

One out of every six American men will develop prostate cancer, and thousands die from this disease every year. Fortunately, keeping your prostate healthy may be as easy as adding flaxseed to your diet.

A recent study, funded by the National Institutes of Health and led by Duke University researchers, found that taking flaxseed supplements before prostate surgery slowed the growth of tumors. Men in the study took 30 grams of flaxseed per day, ground into powdered form and sprinkled on food and drink, for about 30 days before their surgery. Whether the men stuck to a low-fat diet or not, those who took flaxseed had slower growing tumors than those who did not.

Flaxseed has two key ingredients that make it a successful cancer fighter — omega-3 fatty acids and lignans. Researchers suspect omega-3 slows the spread of cancer cells by changing the way cancer cells clump together or stick to other healthy cells. Lignans, fiber-related compounds that act as antioxidants, may work by cutting off a tumor's blood supply and stunting its growth.

For more information on the benefits of omega-3, see the Omega-3 fatty acids chapter.

Whatever the reasons for flaxseed's success, it could be an important part of a healthy diet. Scientists now plan to study if flaxseed can prevent a recurrence of prostate cancer or even help healthy men avoid prostate cancer in the first place.

2 terrific ways to help your head

Flaxseed is a wonder in more ways than one. Just look at how it helps your head, both inside and out.

Manages migraines. Eating certain foods can trigger migraines, but adding some flaxseed to your diet may help relieve them. That's because the omega-3 fatty acids in flaxseed ease inflammation of the blood vessels in your brain. They may also protect nerves. Studies have shown that fish oil supplements, also rich in omega-3 fatty acids, can help people have fewer and less intense migraines. Flaxseed is a tastier way to achieve the same effect. A daily tablespoon of ground flaxseed should do the trick.

Beautifies hair. Even if you don't have flaxen hair, you can give your hair a boost with flaxseed. Rich in omega-3 fatty acids, flaxseeds provide the nutrients your hair follicles need. For beautiful, healthy, dandruff-free hair, aim for four to six tablespoons of ground flaxseed per day. Just sprinkle some in your yogurt, cereal, or salad. Flaxseed oil can also keep your hair and scalp healthy.

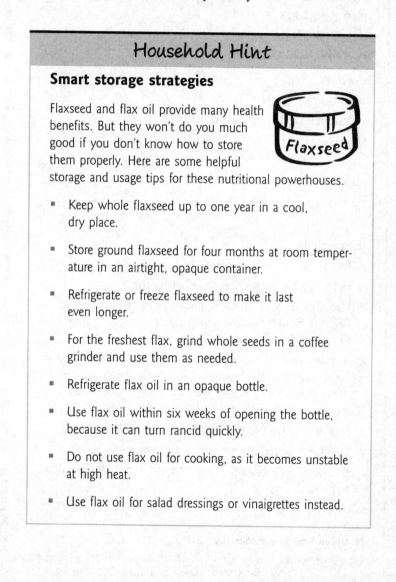

Household Hint

Smart storage strategies

Flaxseed and flax oil provide many health benefits. But they won't do you much good if you don't know how to store them properly. Here are some helpful storage and usage tips for these nutritional powerhouses.

- Keep whole flaxseed up to one year in a cool, dry place.

- Store ground flaxseed for four months at room temperature in an airtight, opaque container.

- Refrigerate or freeze flaxseed to make it last even longer.

- For the freshest flax, grind whole seeds in a coffee grinder and use them as needed.

- Refrigerate flax oil in an opaque bottle.

- Use flax oil within six weeks of opening the bottle, because it can turn rancid quickly.

- Do not use flax oil for cooking, as it becomes unstable at high heat.

- Use flax oil for salad dressings or vinaigrettes instead.

Flaxseed Cornbread

Ingredients

1 1/3 cups water

2 Tbsp ground flaxseed

1 cup all-purpose white flour

1 cup cornmeal

4 tsp baking powder

1/3 cup nonfat dry milk powder

3/4 tsp salt

1/4 cup sugar

1/4 cup canola oil

1/4 cup pecans, chopped

Instructions

1. Preheat oven to 425 degrees.
2. Lightly grease an 8-inch-square baking pan.
3. Place 1/3 cup of water in a small saucepan and bring to a boil. Add the ground flaxseed and stir over medium-high heat until thickened. Remove from heat and cool.
4. In a separate bowl, combine flour, cornmeal, baking powder, sugar, dry milk powder and salt, and mix thoroughly. Add the flaxseed mixture, 1 cup of water, and canola oil to dry ingredients. Mix until most of the lumps are smooth.
5. Pour the batter into the greased pan.
6. Sprinkle chopped pecans over the batter.
7. Bake for 20-25 minutes or until an inserted toothpick comes out clean.

(Serves 9)

Nutrition Summary by Serving

225.1 Calories (88.7 calories from fat, 39.40 percent of total); 9.9 g Fats; 4.8 g Protein; 30.6 g Carbohydrates; 0.9 mg Cholesterol; 2.3 g Fiber; 451.1 mg Sodium

Garlic

Amazing herb helps your heart

Garlic does more than make your food taste better. It's also a natural way to lower cholesterol, reduce your blood pressure, and fight heart disease. You might say this common herb is a lifesaver. Here's what it can do for your heart.

Attack atherosclerosis. In lab tests, garlic blocks key enzymes involved in cholesterol synthesis. It also blocks the oxidation of low-density lipoprotein (LDL), or bad cholesterol. If you can stop LDL from becoming oxidized, it does not become as much of a threat to your arteries.

Promising lab results don't always translate into real life. But many studies show that garlic lowers cholesterol, especially in people with high cholesterol who took aged garlic extract or garlic powder. An examination of several positive studies determined that garlic reduced LDL cholesterol by an average of 11.4 percent and total cholesterol and triglycerides by an average of 9.9 percent. In a recent Iranian study, garlic tablets also boosted HDL, or good cholesterol, by 15.7 percent. Garlic also slashed total cholesterol by 12.1 percent and LDL cholesterol by 17.3 percent.

Not all studies support garlic's cholesterol-lowering effects. In fact, a recent government-funded study found that garlic, whether eaten raw in sandwiches or taken in pill form, had no significant effect on LDL cholesterol. Researchers point out that garlic may still have other heart-healthy properties.

Bring down blood pressure. Garlic may also have a positive effect on your blood pressure. In six studies, garlic lowered blood pressure. However, other studies found no such benefit. Even if garlic does not directly reduce blood pressure, it can serve as a tasty substitute for salt in flavoring your food. Cutting back on sodium is one way to keep your blood pressure under control.

Hammer heart disease. Besides its potential to lower cholesterol and blood pressure, garlic may provide other benefits to your heart. Thanks to its antioxidant powers, garlic may help reduce oxidative stress, which can lead to heart disease. Garlic has been reported to reduce unstable angina and increase the elasticity of your blood vessels.

Recent studies also show that it can slow the progression of coronary artery calcification, or hardening of the arteries, in people taking statins. Garlic can also control your levels of homocysteine. High levels of this amino acid can predict heart disease. When you add more garlic to your diet, you protect your heart in a variety of ways.

Crush blood clots with garlic

Blood clots can trigger heart attacks and strokes, but they are no match for garlic. This common herb prevents blood clots and improves circulation. The organosulfur compounds in garlic, including allicin, stop platelets from clumping together and forming clots. Studies using various forms of garlic, including garlic powder, garlic oil, and aged garlic extract, have found that garlic works for both healthy people and those with heart disease.

Raw garlic works best, since heat can rob garlic of its anti-clotting compounds. But a recent study found that when you crush garlic before cooking it, the garlic loses less of its powers. You can always make up for what you lose by eating more garlic. If you take warfarin or other blood thinners, you may want to limit your garlic intake.

Garlic slashes cancer risk

A healthy diet, rich in fiber from fruits, vegetables, and whole grains and low in red meat and processed foods, can help prevent colon cancer. Regular screenings are important, too. But, if you're looking for an edge to beat this dreaded disease, wake up and smell the garlic. This fragrant herb inhibits cancer growth and reduces your cancer risk. Italian researchers found that people who ate the most garlic had a 26-percent lower risk of colon cancer compared to those who ate the least. Even moderate garlic consumption made a difference.

This study does not stand alone. A recent Japanese study found that garlic halts the spread of pre-cancerous lesions in the colon. And a review of all studies over the past 10 years found "consistent scientific evidence" that garlic reduces the risk of colon cancer. Eating more garlic may also drastically lower your risk of other cancers, including those of the mouth, throat, and kidneys.

Garlic gets its anti-cancer powers mainly from its organosulfur compounds, which inhibit tumor growth. In addition to these compounds, garlic's selenium content also plays a role in fighting cancer. How much selenium garlic has depends on the soil in which it's grown. Selenium-enriched garlic fights cancer even better than regular garlic, according to one study.

To get the anti-cancer benefits of garlic, many experts recommend aiming for two to four cloves of fresh, minced garlic each day. You can also take garlic in supplement form. Shoot for 600 milligrams (mg) to 1,200 mg of aged garlic extract or take two 200-mg freeze-dried garlic tablets three times daily. Make sure the tablets are standardized to 1.3 percent allicin or 0.6 percent allicin. Here's another helpful tip — don't cook garlic immediately after peeling it. Let it sit for about 15 minutes, then cook it briefly. This will help preserve its cancer-fighting benefits.

Flavorful way to fight food poisoning

Garlic doesn't just make your food tastier — it makes your food safer, too. That's because garlic can banish bacteria that cause food poisoning. Raw garlic has long been known for its antibacterial properties, but a recent New Mexico State University study found that cooked garlic can help, too. The study tested garlic against common foodborne bacteria, such as *salmonella*, *listeria*, and *shigella*. Both raw and boiled garlic extracts were added to bacteria growing in lab dishes and in a nutrient broth. Raw garlic killed about twice as many bacteria in the lab dishes and about 10 times more in the broth, but cooked garlic still retained some of its antibacterial powers.

Bulb boosts immune system

Eat more garlic, and you'll get fewer colds. According to a British study, this super kitchen staple can fight infection and keep your immune system in tiptop shape. In the study, 146 people took either a garlic supplement or a placebo for 12 weeks between November and February, prime cold season. During that time, those who took garlic were less likely to catch a cold. Even if they caught a cold, it did not last as long, and they were less likely to catch another one, which suggests garlic strengthens the immune system. Garlic even helped reduce the seriousness of symptoms like sneezing, coughing, and runny nose. What's more, you don't have to go overboard. Just one capsule a day did the trick.

You can also get your garlic the old-fashioned way — through food. Chicken soup is one old folk remedy that scientists say really works — and at least part of its success comes from garlic, which boasts anti-microbial powers and relieves congestion. The compound allicin gives garlic its cold-fighting powers.

When you have a cold, you're often sick and tired. Garlic may help restore some of your pep. Studies show garlic may fight fatigue in a variety of ways. In animal studies, it boosts exercise endurance. In people, garlic helps with the fatigue that comes with a cold. It also works for physical fatigue and general weariness.

Dodge diabetes with garlic

As diabetes becomes more widespread, dietary changes become even more important. When it comes to preventing or managing this common condition, every little bit helps. If you're worried about diabetes, reach for some garlic. Garlic may lower blood sugar, cholesterol, and triglycerides — all key factors in diabetes.

A recent Kuwait study of rats found that high doses of garlic significantly lowered blood glucose, or blood sugar. Garlic also lowered cholesterol by 11 to 14 percent and triglcyerides, dangerous fats in the blood, by 38 percent. Raw garlic worked better than boiled garlic in the study, especially for lowering blood sugar. These promising results could apply to people, as well. In fact, several studies have shown that raw garlic cloves lower fasting blood sugar in both people and animals.

As usual, the sulfur compound allicin holds the key to garlic's success. Experts suspect allicin works by competing with insulin for insulin-inactivating sites in the liver. This results in an increase of free insulin to keep glucose in check. Garlic's sulfur compounds may also directly or indirectly stimulate the secretion of insulin from the pancreas. Simply adding more garlic to your diet may help you avoid both diabetes and heart disease. Aim for 4 grams of fresh garlic, or about four cloves, or 8 milligrams of essential oil each day.

Surprising way to treat UTIs

You probably know drinking cranberry juice helps treat or prevent urinary tract infections. But when it comes to fighting UTIs, garlic is no slouch. Like cranberry juice, garlic destroys bacteria in the urinary tract. Garlic's antibiotic powers work against organisms that commonly cause UTIs, including *E. coli*, *Proteus* species, *Klebsiella*, and *staphylococcal* and *streptococcal* species.

Make room for more garlic in your diet. Two to three cloves of freshly chopped garlic a day should do the trick. For more flavor, combine the garlic with olive oil and cook it. You can also take garlic supplements. Just make sure the odor component is not removed, since that's what gives garlic its antibacterial action. Enteric-coated garlic capsules combined with chlorophyll help reduce odor.

Household Hint

Repel pests with garlic

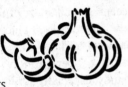

The wonderful smell of garlic cooking can draw a crowd in your kitchen. Fortunately for your garden, garlic isn't as tempting to deer, insects, and mites. You can use this fragrant herb to keep garden pests away.

- Plant garlic between rows of vegetables or near roses, raspberries, and fruit trees. Garlic keeps aphids away from roses, red spiders away from tomatoes, and Japanese beetles away from raspberries. It also repels weevils, carrot flies, moles, and fruit tree borers.

- Dust some garlic powder directly on your plants.

- Spray your plants. Some commercial deer repellents use garlic as an active ingredient, but you can make your own garlic spray. Just blend six cloves of garlic, an onion, and one tablespoon each of cayenne pepper and biodegradable dishwasher liquid. Add a quart of water, let it steep for 24 hours, and strain.

Ginger

Take a detour from queasy street

Riding in the car, you feel sick to your stomach, you're sweating, your heart is racing, and you're having trouble breathing. Sounds like you have motion sickness.

The tiny bones and fluid-filled tubes in your inner ear tell your brain your position in space, but sometimes your senses can play tricks on you. Motion sickness happens when your eyes and your ears are sending your brain different messages. It can occur when you ride in a car, train, boat, or airplane or when you give your body other types of thrills, like watching an IMAX movie or riding the Tilt-A-Whirl.

But you can get help from an old-time remedy — ginger. The part of the ginger plant you eat is often called "ginger root," but it's not really a root. It's the rhizome, or underground stem, of the ginger plant. The lovely scent comes from gingerols, phytochemicals — natural plant chemicals — that give it the power to quell nausea. In fact, one study found ginger works better than the anti-nausea drug dimenhydrinate (Dramamine) at fighting motion sickness.

Ginger helps you feel better three ways:

- blocks chemical receptors in your stomach to relieve nausea

- dilates blood vessels to create a warming effect

- works as an antioxidant to battle free radicals

Ginger may also fight other kinds of nausea. People who get chemotherapy treatment for cancer often feel nauseous, and research shows taking ginger may help. Another study found taking at least

1 gram of ginger — that's just half a teaspoon — helped stave off the nausea and vomiting that often follow surgery.

Drinking ginger tea when you feel sick to your stomach really works. You can brew up a big batch using one-half cup of sliced, fresh ginger and six cups of water. Let it simmer for 20 minutes, and sweeten with honey if you wish. Ginger may cause digestive woes, like heartburn, diarrhea, and mouth irritation, but that's rare.

Household Hint

Fresh is best

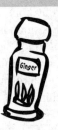

Ginger is available dried and powdered in the spice section of your supermarket, fresh in the produce section, and packaged in supplements. It's also an ingredient in gingersnap cookies and in drinks like ginger tea and ginger ale. Check the labels of packaged ginger foods to be sure they're made from real ginger. For the highest levels of natural plant chemicals that provide ginger's health benefits, buy the fresh root and take it home to chop yourself.

Fight dangerous inflammation with ginger

Almost 100,000 tons of ginger are produced around the world each year. Although it's used primarily as a culinary spice, this popular plant has incredible healing powers.

Ginger "snaps" at arthritis pain. Take a pinch of ginger instead of a daily pain reliever, and you may find yourself forgetting you even have arthritis. Experts think natural substances in ginger called gingerols reduce inflammation by chasing down free radicals before they can damage your joints. Ginger also stops cells in your joints from pumping out cytokines and chemokines — natural chemicals that cause inflammation.

One study found gingerols do their job similar to the COX-2 inhibiting drugs that may already be in your medicine cabinet, like celecoxib (Celebrex). These drugs work by blocking a natural enzyme, cyclooxygenase-2 (COX-2), which brings on inflammation. By stopping COX-2, ginger stops the pain and swelling that make arthritis such a burden on your body. People with knee pain from arthritis had relief from taking about two teaspoons of diced, fresh ginger twice each day.

Ginger may also fight pain and inflammation when you rub it directly on your painful joints. You can buy topical ginger creams, like ZingiberRx Joint and Muscle Cream, to soothe muscle and joint pain. The natural chemicals in ginger can migrate through your skin, making these creams effective pain relievers.

Ginger in supplement form acts as a blood thinner. Taking it may increase the effects of blood-thinning drugs like warfarin (Coumadin). Talk to your doctor before you combine the two.

Spice up your cancer defense. The phytochemicals in ginger may also battle some kinds of cancer. Ginger's power to fight inflammation gets the credit. Ginger's antioxidants help fight ovarian cancer, a deadly disease that affects more than 20,000 women every year. Antioxidants do the job in two ways:

- leading cancer cells to commit suicide, a process known as apoptosis

- encouraging cancer cells to digest or attack themselves, referred to as autophagy

Repeated chemotherapy treatments can make the cancer cells resistant to apoptosis. With ginger, this doesn't happen. Ginger promotes autophagy, as well as apoptosis, making it a powerful weapon against ovarian cancer cells. In fact, in one study, ginger killed cancer cells better than the chemotherapy drugs usually used.

Pineapple Ginger Salsa

Ingredients

30 oz pineapple chunks,
    canned in juice, drained

2 Tbsp sugar

2 tsp fresh ginger root,
    peeled and minced

3/4 cup water

2 tsp lemon juice

I tsp distilled white vinegar

Instructions

1. Mix pineapple chunks, sugar, minced ginger root, and 3/4 cup of water in a saucepan.

2. Bring mixture to a boil over medium-high heat. Reduce heat and simmer, stirring often, until pineapple is soft. Add more water if needed. Cook for 20-30 minutes.

3. Remove from heat and add lemon juice, vinegar, and salt and pepper to taste. Refrigerate until ready to serve.

(Serves 6)

Nutrition Summary by Serving

102.4 Calories (1.4 calories from fat, 1.41 percent of total); 0.2 g Fats; 0.7 g Protein; 26.5 g Carbohydrates; 0.0 mg Cholesterol; 1.9 g Fiber; 8.6 mg Sodium

Goji berry

Ancient Chinese superfruit protects your vision

There's a new berry in town, and its name is goji. Actually, goji berry is not new at all. People in China have been eating it for centuries to help them live longer and stay healthy.

Also called wolfberry, the goji is a small, bright red berry that some people say tastes like a cross between a cherry and a cranberry. But it's still so new to the United States that little is known about the fruit's benefits. In fact, the U.S. Department of Agriculture has not yet analyzed the nutritional content of goji berry. But researchers have started looking at the concentrated nutrients in goji, finding a whopping number of antioxidants like zeaxanthin, beta carotene, vitamin C, and zinc.

That high level of antioxidants is what makes goji the berry that may protect your vision. Here's how it works.

- Cataracts, or cloudy areas of the eye lens that block vision, are one of the most common vision problems in people older than 50. They may be related to how much vitamin C you get. That's because vitamin C may help protect your eyes against damaging free radicals. Researchers in Japan found middle-aged people with diets high in vitamin C had a lower risk of developing cataracts than people who got less of this important vitamin. Dried goji berries have about the same level of vitamin C as fresh lemons, so you can get half your daily requirement in just 2 ounces of goji.

- Age-related macular degeneration (AMD) is another common problem of older eyes. AMD occurs because of damage to the macula, or the center part of the retina at the back of your eye. It's kind of like having a black spot in the center of the movie screen that should reflect images from your eye's lens. The retina is especially prone to free-radical damage because of its exposure to light and oxygen. Antioxidants — specifically beta carotene, vitamin C, vitamin E, and zinc — may stop this damage. Goji berries have at least three of the four antioxidants in this protective cocktail of nutrients.

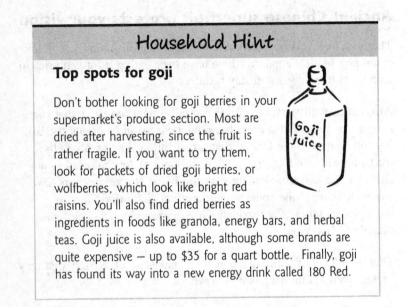

Household Hint

Top spots for goji

Don't bother looking for goji berries in your supermarket's produce section. Most are dried after harvesting, since the fruit is rather fragile. If you want to try them, look for packets of dried goji berries, or wolfberries, which look like bright red raisins. You'll also find dried berries as ingredients in foods like granola, energy bars, and herbal teas. Goji juice is also available, although some brands are quite expensive — up to $35 for a quart bottle. Finally, goji has found its way into a new energy drink called 180 Red.

Stay young with goji power

Advertisements for goji juice are full of promises and hype, making claims that it's the most nutritious food in the world, it makes your muscles stronger, or it works like a natural Viagra. Some of that is likely exaggeration. But the tiny goji berry can make you feel younger physically and mentally, according to recent studies.

Increases energy. First, researchers tested how goji polysaccharides — complex carbohydrates in goji berry — help muscles recover from exhausting exercise. They found that mice in a program of vigorous exercise for 30 days benefited from these special goji carbs. The compounds helped antioxidant enzymes in their muscles battle the stress caused by overuse. That makes goji a great food to help you feel better after exercise.

Other scientists looked at how drinking goji juice may help you feel better mentally and physically. For two weeks people in the study drank about half a cup of goji juice every day. Most reported they had more energy, slept better, were mentally sharper, and generally felt more content. They also reported better athletic performance and digestive regularity.

Slows down aging. These results make goji berry sound like a fountain of youth, and in fact the fruit has that reputation. One region of China where goji berries have been grown and eaten for 2,000 years is known for its long-living population, with 16 times as many people of 100 years or older as the rest of China. There's also the legend of Li Qing Yuen, a Chinese man said to have lived to be 252 years old — simply by eating goji every day.

Just exactly what is so great about goji? It has lots of antioxidants, including loads of zeaxanthin and about as much vitamin C as the same amount of fresh lemon. Those special polysaccharides in goji are believed to slow the effects of aging on your eyes, brain, and many other cells in the body. Finally, goji is said to encourage your pituitary gland to secrete human growth hormone, which some people think slows the signs of aging. So try goji for some extra "get up and go."

Goji is "berry" good, but it's not for everyone. Talk to your doctor first if you take a blood thinner. You should also avoid goji berry if you are getting radiation therapy. And beware of the fruit if you're allergic to other members of the nightshade family, like eggplant or tomatoes.

Quickie Oatmeal Crunch

Ingredients

1/2 cup margarine
3/4 cup brown sugar, packed
1 tsp vanilla extract
1/2 tsp baking soda
2 cups rolled oats
1/2 cup raisins
1/2 cup dried goji berries, chopped

Instructions

1. Preheat oven to 350°F, and grease a 9x13-inch baking pan.
2. In large skillet, melt margarine and brown sugar.
3. Remove from heat and stir in the remaining ingredients.
4. Spread into pan and bake for 15-20 minutes. Cool; cut into squares.

(Serves 24)

Nutrition Summary by Serving

96.5 Calories (38.2 calories from fat, 39.58 percent of total); 4.2 g Fats; 1.2 g Protein; 14.0 g Carbohydrates; 0.0 mg Cholesterol; 0.8 g Fiber; 80.6 mg Sodium

Green tea

Nip cavities in the bud

Drink a few cups of green tea and you could avoid dentists drills and bills. That may sound too good to be true, but scientists say green tea hounds cavity-causing bacteria at every turn. The first troublemakers required for cavities are bacteria like the *Streptococcus mutans* (*S. mutans*) and *Streptococcus sobrinus* naturally found in your mouth. The good news is studies show the catechins in tea can inhibit these bacteria and even kill them. The surviving *S. mutans* and their buddies want to stick to your teeth, but they need help from an enzyme called glucosyltransferase to do it. The catechins in green tea also inhibit this enzyme.

If the bacteria find a way to stick to your teeth, they become part of a film called plaque. That's when the bacteria start churning out acid that eats into your teeth and causes cavities. But the bacteria need sugars to make all this happen. That sugar mostly comes from food sugars, which is why dentists tell you to eat less of them. But even if you give up sugar, an enzyme called amylase can convert starchy foods into sugars *S. mutans* can use. Fortunately for you, green tea compounds inhibit amylase as well.

Human studies suggest people who drink unsweetened green tea develop fewer cavities and what few they do get are less severe. Combine this easy cavity killer with brushing, flossing, and wise eating and you might never get another cavity.

Drink up to keep blood sugar down

One reason diabetes develops is because your body's own personal version of "Jeeves the butler" goes missing and can't do his job. Fortunately, a few cups of green tea may bring him back so he can help you avoid diabetes — or at least fend off its complications.

Like the British manors of the 1920s, many of your cells have a kind of "Jeeves." Take your fat cells, for example. They create a protein called GLUT-4 that meets visitors at the "door" and determines whether to let them in. Insulin and glucose (blood sugar) are frequent visitors because your cells need glucose for energy, and insulin helps them get it. Usually your GLUT-4 escorts the glucose right in. That helps lower the amount of glucose in your bloodstream so you're less likely to get diabetes — and less likely to get worse if you already have it.

Animal studies suggest that a high-fat or high-sugar diet can keep your cells from making GLUT-4 — which means it can't answer the door when glucose comes knocking. Without a place to go, the glucose builds up in your bloodstream. Fortunately, scientists from Taiwan discovered that animals fed green tea along with their chow developed lower blood sugar than animals who drank water. They also found signs that green tea raises the number of GLUT-4 proteins available and helps glucose get into cells. With GLUT-4 back on the job, you're less likely to get diabetes and more likely to keep your blood sugar levels down.

But don't think that's all green tea can do for you. If you already have diabetes, your risk of complications, like cataracts, automatically goes up. Fortunately, a University of Scranton animal study suggests green tea can help. Researchers discovered that drinking four or five cups of green tea lowers blood sugar, which helps inhibit the cataract-forming process.

Experts say more research is needed before they can comfortably recommend green tea for diabetes. But if you're worried about getting diabetes — or even if you already have it — why not try drinking some green tea every day? You might prevent or even reverse diabetes with this popular brew. Start small to see how the caffeine in this drink may affect you. If it keeps you awake at night or makes you nervous, cut back or switch to decaffeinated green tea.

Sip a summer skin saver

Drinking green tea isn't like putting a bodyguard between you and skin cancer — it's like having a whole team of them. If scientists are right, the polyphenols in green tea may help your skin wield an arsenal of weapons against the sun damage that triggers skin cancer.

The secret may be green tea's polyphenols, suggests a study from the University of Alabama at Birmingham. The study found that animals weathered ultraviolet-B radiation better if they drank water laced with green tea polyphenols. Here are just a few examples of how polyphenols protected them.

- They had fewer tumors, and the tumors they did have were smaller.

- They produced fewer compounds linked to the growth and spread of cancer.

- They made less of two compounds that help tumors develop blood vessels. Tumor blood vessels not only bring nourishment to the tumors but may also help them grow.

- They made more cells that act like pesticides against tumor cells.

But don't think tea can only help animals. A study from Dartmouth Medical School in New Hampshire found that people who drank two or more cups of green or black tea a day for at least a month cut their risk of two types of skin cancer — squamous cell carcinoma and basal cell carcinoma — by 20 to 30 percent.

Don't throw out your sunscreen just yet. Instead, combine tea drinking with regular sunscreen use for best results. And for even more protection, add a lemon wedge to your tea. Studies suggest lemon contributes to the protection people get from drinking tea.

Household Hint

'Neat' way to clean your fireplace

Cleaning out your fireplace can make a mess, but you can fix that. Make a pot of tea, using loose tea leaves. Sprinkle the damp tea leaves over the ashes. When you lift them out, you won't stir up dust clouds, and your floor and furniture will stay clean.

Easy way to keep your memory sharp

Most people in Japan have lower odds of dementia than Europeans and Americans. The Japanese also drink plenty of green tea. Now scientists say the two may be connected. Researchers from Japan's University of Tohoku examined the mental status test results of 1,000 people age 70 and older. The tests assessed mental abilities like memory, attention, and ability to follow instructions. Declines in these abilities are often a symptom of oncoming dementia.

The study participants were also asked which beverages they drank and how often. Those who drank at least two cups of green tea every day had the lowest risk of losing their memory and thinking ability. But even those who drank only four to six cups a week were less likely to show signs of sagging mental powers than people who drank tea three times a week or less.

The Tohoku researchers suggest that catechins in green tea — especially the one called epigallocatechin-3-gallate (EGCG) — may help protect your brain. Experts once thought EGCG's antioxidant abilities helped defend the brain from Alzheimer's, but the Japanese researchers think EGCG may do better than that. They point out that one symptom of Alzheimer's disease is plaques that form in your brain. The main component of these plaques is a protein called beta amyloid that can damage your brain tissue. But EGCG can slip into your brain and may help protect it against beta amyloid and its effects.

The Japanese researchers caution that this study doesn't necessarily prove that green tea can stop dementia. They point out that most Japanese drink their tea as part of social activities — and social activities have also been shown to help protect you from dementia. But don't be discouraged. Results from other studies hint that green tea may still have more to offer than just its thirst-quenching ability. Consider these examples.

- Mice prone to memory problems and brain deterioration were given water, green tea, or oolong tea to drink for four months. The mice who drank tea showed significant improvements in both memory and brain health, say Princeton University researchers.

■ Lab tests at the University of Newcastle upon Tyne in England found that green tea extract inhibits the activities of three enzymes linked to Alzheimer's disease. Although extracts are usually more powerful than regular tea, the study's lead researcher suggests that regular green tea may still help boost memory.

While scientists continue to study the potential of green tea, why not give it a try yourself? Enjoy a cup over breakfast, or share a pot of tea with friends at lunch. You'll enjoy drinking this delicious drink now, and your brain may thank you for years to come.

Pump up the power of antibiotics

Green tea turned 20 percent of drug-resistant superbugs into helpless wimps, report researchers from Egypt's Alexandria University. The same bacteria that had virtually ignored antibiotics before were easily wiped out by a combination of antibiotics and green tea. And that's not all.

The scientists pitted teams of green tea and antibiotics against 28 different disease-causing microbes. No matter which antibiotic they used, green tea pumped up the bacteria-killing powers of the drug and destroyed the bacteria's resistance to antibiotics. So the next time your doctor prescribes an antibiotic, try taking your pills with green tea. You might be pleasantly surprised at the results.

Go green to prevent inflammation

A compound found in soothing green tea could be the key to reducing inflammation, joint damage, and more. The catechins in green tea may not be common treatments for rheumatoid arthritis (RA) or urinary tract infections today, but research hints they may have a role to play in the future.

■ A lab study by the University of Michigan Health System found that a tea catechin called EGCG inhibited two compounds famed for creating the joint damage of rheumatoid arthritis. EGCG also blocked production of a hormone-like substance that helps trigger painful RA inflammation in your joints.

■ Experts from the University of Pittsburgh School of Medicine think green tea may help protect against bladder infections. They found that bladder cells exposed to tea catechins were less likely to become inflamed and die after exposure to hydrogen peroxide, which damages cells. This may mean green tea helps protect your bladder from the inflammation and injury bladder infections and other bladder problems can cause. Scientists say more research about inflammation and green tea is coming soon, so stay tuned.

Latest scoop on tea and prostate cancer

Don't believe everything you read. A 2006 study found that drinking green tea makes no difference in your risk of prostate cancer — yet, a newer study disagrees. Here's what you need to know.

At first, the original 2006 study seemed bulletproof. This Japanese study of 19,000 found that men who drank five cups of tea daily were no less likely to die of prostate cancer than men who drank a single cup. But a newer study from Japan's National Cancer Center followed 49,000 men for at least 10 years. This study suggested that green tea may not prevent all prostate cancers, but it may cut your odds of advanced or life-threatening prostate cancer by half. What's more, the more tea the men drank, the lower their risk dropped.

The researchers suspect that one of tea's polyphenols — an antioxidant called EGCG — may fight prostate cancer in several ways. For example, EGCG may trigger the death of cancer cells or slow their growth. It may also take aim at advanced prostate cancer by inhibiting a dangerous compound. Research has linked this compound to aggressive prostate cancer and to the spread of cancer in people who already have prostate cancer.

Turbocharge tea's health benefits

Make lemon your main squeeze when you drink tea and you may get four times as many health-building compounds from your tea. A study from Purdue University found that you only get about 20 percent of tea's healthiest compounds — polyphenols called catechins — when you drink your tea straight. But add a squeeze of lemon juice after your tea brews and that number jumps to 80 percent. Here's why. Extra acidity makes catechins more stable so your body has time to absorb more of them. Lemon juice proved to be the best catechin preserver, the researchers say, but orange juice, lime juice, and grapefruit juice are good second choices.

Before you try this, remember to wash your citrus fruit thoroughly to avoid pesticides and other problems. And be wary of lemon wedges in restaurants. Research shows they may be contaminated with potentially dangerous microbes.

Green Tea Cream Cheese Dip

Ingredients

1 cup brewed green tea,
    use 3 green tea bags
1 cup low-fat cream cheese
2 Tbsp fresh basil,
    finely minced

Instructions

1. Heat 1 cup of water to a boil and allow to cool for 1 minute.

2. Pour hot water over 3 green tea bags and allow to steep for 3 to 5 minutes.

3. Drain bags and remove from water.

4. Allow tea to cool to room temperature or cool in the refrigerator, covered, until ready to use.

5. Add cream cheese and fresh basil in a blender and blend on medium-high speed until smooth. Gradually add tea liquid until the mixture is the desired consistency.

6. Refrigerate, covered, for at least one hour. Use as a spread on bagels, crackers, or as a dip for vegetables and chips.

(Serves 4)

Nutrition Summary By Serving

139.6 Calories (95.1 calories from fat, 68.16 percent of total); 10.6 g Fats; 6.4 g Protein; 4.4 g Carbohydrates; 33.6 mg Cholesterol; 0.1 g Fiber; 179.4 mg Sodium

Honey

Discover the healing wonder of honey

Eat honey, my son, for it is good, was King Solomon's advice thousands of years ago. Now today's researchers are finding out just how wise Solomon was.

Tell a cough to get lost. A study of sick children aged 2 to 18 discovered that those who took honey before bedtime coughed less and slept better than kids who took an over-the-counter cough syrup. The researchers chose buckwheat honey because dark honeys have more antioxidants than lighter ones. But honey may also work because it is a demulcent, a soother that gently coats irritated areas to ease inflammation. That's why it feels so good when you have a sore throat. That same soothing power may also help honey halt a cough.

This sweet, inexpensive cure isn't just for kids, so try it the next time you get sick. Or turn to a mixture of two teaspoons of honey in a cup of warm pineapple juice to silence your cough. A few teaspoons of lemon juice and honey in warm water or hot tea will also provide comforting relief. Just remember, never give honey to children under age 1. Doctors say it could put them at risk for botulism.

Get your system moving. Smooth, sweet-tasting honey is an age-old Greek remedy for constipation, and scientists say it really works.

A small Greek study found that people were more likely to get loose stools within 10 hours of taking 1 1/2 tablespoons of honey. The researchers suspect the sugars in honey may be responsible. Like many other foods, honey contains the sugars fructose and glucose. That's sweet news since your body needs glucose to help it absorb fructose. However, some people can't absorb all the fructose in honey, and scientists think the unabsorbed fructose travels to the colon where bacteria ferment it. This produces substances that may help speed up your bowel processes so you can get back to normal.

While this remedy may not work for everyone, it's worth a try. Stir one to three tablespoons of honey into a glass of warm water, and drink up. This honey potion is far more pleasant than laxatives, and it may bring you just as much relief.

Solve a hidden cause of tummy trouble

You just had toast with honey and now you have bloating, gassiness, and stomach pain. Maybe you even have diarrhea. If this is a regular problem for you, you may have dietary fructose intolerance.

This condition, also called fructose malabsorption, occurs because your body does a poor job digesting fructose, a kind of sugar found in many foods. The sugar glucose can help your body digest fructose, but only if the food contains at least as much of the first sugar as the second. Honey contains more fructose than glucose, so it's particularly hard for people with this problem to digest.

If you suspect you have dietary fructose intolerance, ask your doctor to test you for it. You will need to avoid such foods as honey, apples, pears, apple juice, and anything sweetened with high fructose corn syrup, like soft drinks. Fructose hides in many other foods and drinks as well, so your best bet is to work with a doctor or dietitian to build a diet that will make you feel better.

Beat insomnia with this sleeper hit

You're so tired that the very thought of Sleeping Beauty or Rip Van Winkle makes you jealous. If you can't get to sleep, can't stay asleep, or just sleep poorly, you may have insomnia. And honey just may be your ticket back to dreamland. It may not sound like a potent remedy, but it has two surprisingly effective secret weapons.

Glucose. When this sugar gets in your body, it triggers a chain reaction that feeds the sleep chemical, tryptophan, to your brain. The tryptophan is converted to serotonin and then to melatonin. Both compounds help you relax and fall asleep so you're less likely to lie awake staring at the ceiling.

Fructose. Together the fructose and glucose in honey help your liver produce glycogen. This glycogen is vital to your brain. In fact, if your brain senses a glycogen shortage, it immediately triggers the release of stress hormones like cortisol and adrenalin. This makes it tougher for you to stay asleep and sleep soundly. Fortunately, an evening dose of honey may supply enough fructose and glucose to help your liver make glycogen all night long. When the brain doesn't run out of glycogen, it doesn't crank up your stress hormones. So you may finally be able to sleep tight throughout the night.

If you'd like to try this honey cure, just take a tablespoon or two an hour before you want to sleep. It may be all you need to put your sleep problems to rest for good.

Heal your body inside and out

A new wound dressing saturated with Manuka honey is so effective the United States military used it to treat burns in Iraq. This "MediHoney" dressing also helps treat wounds in New Zealand, Australia, and Great Britain and can even help prevent infections by antibiotic-resistant bacteria. Best of all, MediHoney is now available in the United States.

Experts say all types of honey have some healing power, but Manuka happens to have a mighty bacteria fighter other honeys lack. But that's not the whole story. When Manuka was pitted against another honey, it tested better against some of the scariest bacteria like *E. coli* and antibiotic-resistant *Staphylococcus aureus.* Yet both honeys stopped the growth of seven types of infectious bacteria — even when the researchers used a solution that was only 11 percent honey.

Perhaps this sweet liquid works so well because it revs up wound healing in five different ways:

- fights infection by pulling vital moisture away from bacteria

- provides a sugar-loaded environment that's tough for bacteria to grow in

- helps reduce inflammation

- generates just enough hydrogen peroxide to serve as a mild antiseptic but not enough to kill your cells

- draws fluid from the wound to help the damaged area clean itself out

Unfortunately, medical professionals strongly recommend against using honey from your pantry for cuts and burns. For one thing, store-bought honey is weaker than the honey used in medical studies. That's because it has been heat-treated, a process that cripples its ability to fend off harmful germs.

Raw honey from the beekeeper's hives has never been heat-treated, so it retains its powers. However, some raw honey also isn't filtered. As a result, impurities may still be present, and you'll get a less sterile product to

Honey can help you beat bad breath, according to a South American folk remedy. To make this honey of a mouthwash, mix a pinch of cinnamon and a teaspoon of honey into hot water. Let cool, then gargle. Use this every morning for fresh breath all day.

put on a wound. So if you try honey, find a beekeeper who offers raw, filtered honey. If you can't find one, check your local drugstore, or call Derma Sciences, Inc., the company that makes MediHoney, at 800-445-7627.

Household Hint

Discover a royal secret for beautiful skin

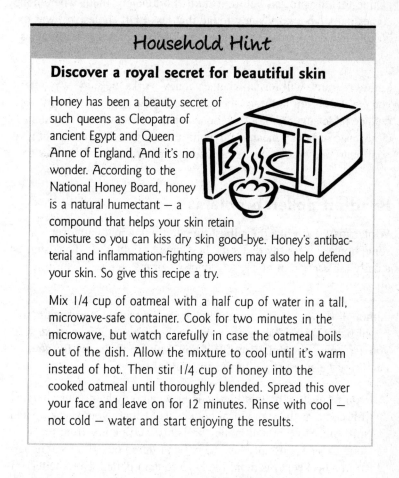

Honey has been a beauty secret of such queens as Cleopatra of ancient Egypt and Queen Anne of England. And it's no wonder. According to the National Honey Board, honey is a natural humectant — a compound that helps your skin retain moisture so you can kiss dry skin good-bye. Honey's antibacterial and inflammation-fighting powers may also help defend your skin. So give this recipe a try.

Mix 1/4 cup of oatmeal with a half cup of water in a tall, microwave-safe container. Cook for two minutes in the microwave, but watch carefully in case the oatmeal boils out of the dish. Allow the mixture to cool until it's warm instead of hot. Then stir 1/4 cup of honey into the cooked oatmeal until thoroughly blended. Spread this over your face and leave on for 12 minutes. Rinse with cool — not cold — water and start enjoying the results.

Guard your heart with a simple switch

Exciting new research from the University of Illinois hints that choosing honey over sugar might help prevent heart attacks. The researchers tested several types of honey to find out which ones might affect your "bad" LDL cholesterol. But they weren't trying to lower cholesterol. Instead, they wanted to keep it from oxidizing. Why? The oxidation of LDL cholesterol helps trigger artery-clogging plaque. Since this plaque can lead to heart attacks, you definitely want to stop the plaque-making process before it starts. Fortunately, that's where honey comes in. A laboratory study found that less LDL cholesterol was oxidized when dark honey was added to blood samples. Lighter honeys weren't as effective.

Future research will reveal whether honey works the same way after you eat it as it did in these laboratory tests. But meanwhile, why not replace table sugar with a dark honey such as buckwheat? The delicious taste of honey means you won't miss sugar, and you might give your heart and arteries an extra dose of protection.

Head off pollen problems

Winter may seem like the silliest time to think about hay fever, but some honey-lovers say that's the best time to fight back. They suggest a daily tablespoon of honey to reduce — or even erase — spring allergy symptoms.

Although studies haven't produced any proof that this works, a number of people say it has brought them relief. The trick is to make sure you use honey the right way. So if you'd like to try honey for your hay fever, be sure to avoid these two mistakes.

■ Don't use store bought honey. Honey can only help your allergies if it contains the same local pollens that trigger your sneezing and sniffling. Store-bought honey probably won't come from local sources, and it usually has the pollen filtered out. But local honey from a beekeeper is more likely to contain pollen. Even better, this pollen probably won't make you sneeze because it passes through your digestive system instead of your nose. Yet daily regular exposure to pollen through honey may help your immune system build up a tolerance to the pollen. As a result, that pollen may fail to trigger allergy symptoms the next time you breathe it in.

■ Don't wait until the first tickle of allergies hits you. Some say honey's sweet cure won't work unless you give it plenty of time. So start taking honey at the beginning of winter to give your immune system several months to adjust. Your nose may just thank you come spring.

Honey is usually harmless, but a few people are allergic to it. If you experience any unusual symptoms after using honey, stop taking it.

Natural protection from food poisoning

If you're worried about food safety — and who isn't — here's some good news. Kansas State University researchers have discovered that treating foods with a mix of dark wildflower honey and tea extract decimates the food poisoning bacteria lurking in foods. For example, treating a slice of turkey breast with Jasmine tea extract and wildflower dark honey reduced the amount of dangerous *Listeria* microbes in the meat. When combined with dark wildflower honey, green tea extract has a similar effect. Even better, these honey-tea extracts kept bacterial populations down for up to 14 days in some types of hot dog.

The researchers hope their tests will lead to a "surface wash" that food manufacturers can use to cleanse their products. That could help prevent food poisoning in both meats and ready-to-eat veggies without contaminating your food with harsh chemicals.

Inulin

3 ways inulin protects your colon

Inulin is one fiber you may not be familiar with. It's not new — it's been an ingredient in your onions and garlic forever. But inulin is getting new respect for what it can do to help your digestive system work smoothly and possibly even prevent colon cancer.

Inulin is a natural soluble fiber that's also a sugar. It's in a class of plant compounds called fructans — they store energy as fructose rather than as glucose. Inulin works as a prebiotic, or food for the helpful bacteria that naturally live in your digestive system. Its most common source is chicory root, long used as a coffee substitute.

Inulin does three great things for your digestion.

Super sources of inulin

- ★ chicory
- ★ onions
- ★ bananas
- ★ wheat
- ★ leeks
- ★ garlic
- ★ asparagus
- ★ Jerusalem artichoke

- ■ It makes a clean sweep of constipation. Doctors suggest you get a mixture of soluble and insoluble fiber to keep you regular — 20 to 30 grams a day for senior adults. Like other soluble fibers, inulin forms a gel in your intestines to carry out fatty substances.

- ■ It battles diseases like ulcerative colitis (UC). This is a type of inflammatory bowel disease that causes pain, diarrhea, and blood in the stool because of damage to colon tissues. Inulin seems to help by slowing inflammation in the colon and boosting the power of the helpful bacteria strains that live there.

- ■ It keeps your colon safe from cancer. Lab studies have shown inulin slows the growth of precancerous areas in the colon.

Experts are still working to find out why, but they suspect inulin causes changes in digestive enzymes to help "friendly" gut bacteria like *bifidobacteria* grow and flourish. The changes also cause more dangerous bacteria to be removed from the colon in bowel movements.

Keep the good, send out the bad — and your whole digestive system will be happier and healthier.

Simple sugar fits diabetes diet

The sweet soluble fiber inulin may be just the ticket for controlling blood sugar. This wonder fiber might even be called a miracle food for people with diabetes.

Maintain balanced blood sugar. People with type 2 diabetes need to get a handle on blood sugar, which can get too high after eating. Unlike other sugars, inulin doesn't raise your blood sugar. That's because it's not broken down in the stomach or small intestine. Instead, it moves right through to your colon. Research found that people with and without diabetes who ate inulin had less rise in their blood sugar. The change was likely due to the way inulin slows the absorption of carbohydrates.

Inulin may help your body absorb important minerals like calcium and magnesium. Research shows that taking inulin allows more of these minerals to be absorbed from the food you eat. That's a bonus if you're battling osteo- porosis or other conditions where you need lots of calcium.

Hold the line on cholesterol and triglycerides. Inulin keeps your cholesterol down like other soluble fibers, such as beta glucan in oats. That's because inulin changes the population of bacteria in your intes- tines, which in turn affects how cholesterol is made. Some studies hint that inulin may work better in people with type 2 diabetes than in healthy people. Inulin also helps lower triglycerides, another form of fat in your blood that you need to keep a lid on.

Keep your weight under control. Inulin has a twin among sugar molecules called oligofructose, which does similar things in your body. Researchers have tested both kinds of sugars to see how they affect weight. Both inulin and oligofructose seem to help people eat less and lose weight. It may be that these sugars fill you up faster, or it may be that they change your digestive bacteria to help you lose weight. Yet another theory is that inulin changes the hunger hormones your body produces so you don't feel as hungry.

However it works to balance your blood sugar, cholesterol, and weight, inulin is a good addition to your diabetes diet.

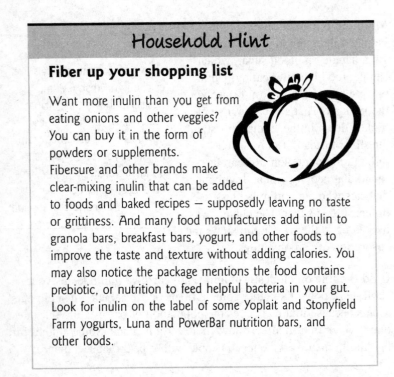

Household Hint

Fiber up your shopping list

Want more inulin than you get from eating onions and other veggies? You can buy it in the form of powders or supplements. Fibersure and other brands make clear-mixing inulin that can be added to foods and baked recipes — supposedly leaving no taste or grittiness. And many food manufacturers add inulin to granola bars, breakfast bars, yogurt, and other foods to improve the taste and texture without adding calories. You may also notice the package mentions the food contains prebiotic, or nutrition to feed helpful bacteria in your gut. Look for inulin on the label of some Yoplait and Stonyfield Farm yogurts, Luna and PowerBar nutrition bars, and other foods.

Leafy greens

4 powerful ways to fend off heart disease

Get back to the basics of good nutrition, and eat what you know you should eat. Spinach — and its many leafy green cousins. Munch on some greens every day to protect your blood vessels and fend off heart disease and stroke.

The category of leafy greens includes more than just iceberg lettuce. Darker, fancier greens — from collards and kale to sorrel and spinach — are more nutritious members of the gang. These powerhouse foods help your heart in four ways.

Ferret out folate. This important B vitamin — called folate in foods like spinach and parsley and folic acid in supplements — may cut your risk of having a stroke by as much as 30 percent. Several studies have shown when people take folic acid, they have lower levels of homocysteine, a marker of heart disease and stroke risk. But experts are debating this chicken-and-egg problem — does homocysteine cause heart problems, or is it just a sign of danger? Either way, it's a fact that the number of strokes has gone down since 1998, when the U.S. government required folic acid to be added to bread and grains.

Count on vitamin K. One cup of fresh kale has more than six times the vitamin K you need in a day. Many seniors don't get enough of this fat-soluble vitamin, but it's important to help your blood clot when you get a

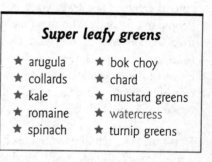

Super leafy greens

- ★ arugula
- ★ collards
- ★ kale
- ★ romaine
- ★ spinach
- ★ bok choy
- ★ chard
- ★ mustard greens
- ★ watercress
- ★ turnip greens

scrape. If you don't get enough, you may raise your risk of hardening of the arteries.

Toss in some "oids." Flavonoids and carotenoids, that is. Leafy green veggies are chock-full of these types of nutrients, and they help protect your heart. One large study found a person's risk of developing cardiovascular disease fell by 11 percent for each daily serving of spinach or other greens eaten.

Make room for minerals. You've probably heard about watching your intake of sodium, or salt, to control blood pressure. Some experts think it's even more important to get plenty of other minerals, including magnesium, potassium, and calcium. That's because these other electrolytes balance out excess salt. Chow down on spinach, kale, and edible seaweed for a great mineral mix.

Keep your memory sharp as a tack

Don't think of forgetfulness as a natural part of getting older. It's not. You can stay mentally alert as you age with a secret weapon in your diet. Here's a hint — it's green, crunchy, and likes to get dressed.

That's right — a nice green salad is your memory's best friend. Researchers at Columbia University found that getting lots of folate, an important B vitamin plentiful in dark greens like spinach and collard greens, may lower your risk of developing Alzheimer's disease. People in this study who fared the best in terms of memory got folate from food as well as folic acid, the man-made form of the vitamin, from supplements. The researchers think low folate levels lead to high levels of homocysteine, an amino acid that may keep DNA from repairing damaged nerve cells. Damaged cells in the brain are more prone to plaque buildup, a sign of Alzheimer's.

But some research hints you must have both folate and vitamin B12 for a truly youthful brain. You'll need to eat about 7 ounces of fresh spinach or turnip greens or 4 ounces of leeks to get the daily recommendation of folate, 400 micrograms. Add a couple ounces of tuna to your salad bowl, and you're good on vitamin B12 as well.

Folate helps you in other important ways:

- A study in the Netherlands found that folic acid supplements slowed hearing loss in aging men and women.

- Getting enough folate, vitamin E, and calcium in your diet may protect you from bacterial vaginosis, a type of vaginal infection. In contrast, eating a high-fat diet may raise your risk of this condition.

Don't go overboard on folic acid

Leafy greens are a great source of folate, a B vitamin that helps your nervous system, protects your heart, and builds DNA in your cells. They're a better choice than supplements. Early research shows that getting too much of this nutrient may encourage cancerous tumors to grow in the colon, prostate, and breast.

The danger may come if you're getting a full day's supply of folic acid — the 400 micrograms (mcg) found in some multivitamins — along with extra folic acid in enriched breads and nutrition bars. Instead, get your folate naturally from veggies. Eating one cup of cooked spinach, collard greens, or turnip greens provides a safe serving of about 170 to 270 mcg.

Household Hint

Eat local for flavor and good health

The average piece of produce travels nearly 1,500 miles before it's eaten in the United States. Now that's changing. You may have heard of the "eat local" movement — people trying to eat food that's grown or produced locally, preferably within 100 miles. These locavores — local eaters — list the benefits.

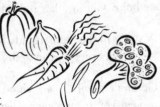

- Produce is fresher, tastier, and may have more nutrients.

- Food may be less prone to contamination. A long journey from another state or nation gives more chances for bacteria to taint food.

- The environment benefits, with less energy used to transport and store food.

- You may pay less due to reduced transport costs. One study found locally grown foods cost an average of $3.80 per pound, while foods from national vendors cost $4.30 per pound.

- You support local farmers, who then help support your town's economy.

Now big supermarkets, including Wal-Mart, A&P, and Hannaford Brothers, are seeking out locally grown produce for their stores. That means you can save even more money by driving to just one location for your food shopping.

2 ways greens keep your body young

Dark leafy greens like Swiss chard, kale, collards, spinach, and turnip greens are great sources of vitamin K. This fat-soluble vitamin, needed to help your blood clot, may also keep your joints and blood vessels youthful.

Older people who get less vitamin K have more problems with osteoarthritis (OA) in their hands and knees. One study found more bone spurs and cartilage loss among people with lower blood levels of this vitamin. That means more pain and swelling in some of the joints you use the most. But that's not all.

Vitamin K in your favorite leafy greens may also fend off varicose veins, those ugly, bulging veins in your legs caused by improper sitting, too much standing, or simply getting older. Researchers found vitamin K activates a protein that keeps your veins healthy. So add some greens to your daily diet, and help keep your body young.

5-a-day plan beats cancer

A big salad for lunch and a serving of greens at dinner can put you well on the path to cancer protection by helping you meet the American Cancer Society's recommendation of five servings of fruits and vegetables a day.

Load up on B vitamins. Studies show certain vitamins that are plentiful in green leafy veggies offer cancer protection. A large survey of several research projects found that lean people who get lots of folate, vitamin B6, and vitamin B12 have a lower risk of developing pancreatic cancer. This deadly cancer is difficult to treat, and experts are still working to figure out exactly what causes it. The study showed these B vitamins had to come from food — not supplements — to be protective.

Similarly, a study in Sweden found that folate, abundant in greens, may protect against breast cancer. Nearly 12,000 postmenopausal women were followed for almost 10 years. Those who took in more folate had a lower risk of developing breast cancer.

Rev up the antioxidants. Researchers in Australia had similar results when they examined squamous cell carcinoma, a type of skin cancer. They found that people who tend to eat lots of fruits and vegetables — especially leafy green veggies — have a lower risk of skin cancer than those who eat more meat and high-fat foods. Antioxidants in the produce, like vitamin C, vitamin E, and lutein, may protect by stopping oxidative damage to cells.

Choose dark over light. Toss up a salad using darker greens to get the most cancer-busting nutrients. Belgian endive and romaine lettuce provide loads of vitamin A and vitamin C, while fresh spinach is a great source of iron, vitamin A, and folate. In contrast, that pale favorite — iceberg lettuce — gives you much less of these vitamins and minerals.

Household Hint

Toss up a tasteful table decoration

Edible table decorations are all the rage, but you don't need to empty your wallet for a lovely arrangement. Browse through your farmers' market for interesting leafy offerings, then arrange them into a tasteful — and tasty — "flower" arrangement for the mantel or dinner table.

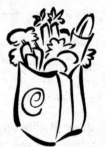

Focus on how the produce looks. Combine colors, like dark spinach leaves with purple cabbage. Look for unusual textures and shapes, such as curly leaf lettuce or ornamental kale. Throw in some asparagus spears for variety. And don't forget about edible flowers, like nasturtiums and violets.

After your dinner party, rinse off the arrangement, chop it into a salad, and enjoy.

Healthy picks from the salad bar

Eating a salad sounds healthy and light, but not all salad bar ingredients are equal. See which greens, veggies, and toppings carry the most nutrition with the least caloric punch.

Poor choice	Healthy substitute	What's the difference?
iceberg lettuce	spinach, romaine lettuce	darker greens have more vitamins
green bell peppers	red, yellow, orange bell peppers	colorful peppers have more vitamin C
artichoke hearts	broccoli, carrots	fewer calories
sun-dried tomatoes	fresh tomatoes	fewer calories, more volume to fill you up
celery sticks	raw or blanched asparagus	more folate
radishes	white mushrooms	good source of minerals and B vitamins
deli-style potato salad, cole slaw	shredded raw veggies like carrots or cabbage	more vitamins, less fat, and fewer calories
raisins, dried cranberries	fresh peaches, pears, or blueberries	fewer calories, more volume to fill you up
croutons	crumbled baked chips	less fat, fewer calories
cracker crumbs	ground flaxseed	good source of omega-3 fatty acids and fiber
creamy ranch or blue cheese salad dressing	oil-and-vinegar salad dressing, heavy on the vinegar	less fat, fewer calories
fat-free salad dressing	reduced-fat salad dressing	a bit of fat helps you absorb nutrients from the veggies
corn oil salad dressing	olive oil or canola oil salad dressing	monounsaturated fats help you absorb antioxidant vitamins from greens
cheddar cheese, blue cheese	mozzarella, goat cheese	less fat
bacon bits	nuts, olives	monounsaturated fats from plant foods are healthier than saturated fats from meat

Enjoy a triple defense against cancer

Greens, glorious greens. They're available year-round, and they can do your colon a world of good. Leafy green vegetables are your triple-strong weapon against colon cancer.

- Fiber in leafy green vegetables can help you reach your goal of getting 25 to 30 grams of fiber a day. Not all experts agree, but fiber may help by keeping digestion regular to flush out cancer-causing toxins.

- Vitamins and phytochemicals, such as folate and isothiocyanates, are abundant in dark greens like spinach, collard greens, and mustard greens. Antioxidant vitamins, in particular, may keep cells safe from the free radical damage that can lead to cancer.

- Weight control is easier if you eat bulky, low-calorie foods like greens. People who are obese have a higher risk of colon cancer. In fact, one study found that men who eat the most produce — two or more servings a day — have an 18 percent lower risk of colon cancer than men who eat fewer servings. Green leafy vegetables offer the most protection.

Go green for a healthy prostate

The more salad on your plate, the younger your prostate.

An enlarged prostate is common in older men, and it may be due to a condition called benign prostatic hyperplasia (BPH). It's an annoyance, causing problems like frequent urination, difficulty urinating, and urinary tract infections.

But there's help. The well-known Health Professionals Follow-Up Study found that men who eat plenty of vegetables and fruit — especially those with lots of beta carotene, lutein, and vitamin C — have a lower chance of developing BPH. Experts think these antioxidants block the inflammation and oxidative stress that occurs with BPH. Kale, spinach, and turnip greens are fabulous leafy choices that contain all three protective nutrients.

What's more, lab studies hint that certain carotenoids — nutrients in leafy greens — may slow the growth of prostate cancer cells. Let's hear a holler for collards.

Lutein & zeaxanthin

Fight vision loss and win

Age-proof your eyes and help stave off vision loss just by eating delicious foods, like leafy greens. These foods help prevent age-related macular degeneration (AMD) and blindness. But even if you already have AMD, you can improve your eyesight without glasses, contact lenses, surgery, drugs, or medicine of any kind.

The secret, of course, is two natural pigments called lutein and zeaxanthin. Not only do they add color to leafy greens, they also fortify your eyes against macular degeneration. In fact, a recent study found that people who got the most lutein and zeaxanthin in their diets were less likely to get "wet" AMD, the kind that can steal your sight in just a few weeks. But that's not the most exciting thing about lutein and zeaxanthin.

A study of 90 people with dry AMD revealed that those who took 10 milligrams (mg) of lutein every day had measurably sharper vision by the end of one year. Experts think lutein and zeaxanthin in the eye may act like a sunscreen against the shorter wavelengths of sunlight. These short wavelengths may help cause AMD.

Although the people in the study took supplements, you can get up to 10 mg of lutein from foods you may already have in your kitchen. In fact, you'll get nearly that much if you boil a half cup of frozen turnip greens and eat them for dinner. Other frozen half-cuppers that can give you at least 10 mg include spinach, kale, and collards.

If you prefer more variety, consider getting some of your lutein from breakfast. Although a hard-boiled egg has less than 1 mg of lutein,

Super sources of lutein/zeaxanthin	
★ eggs	★ spinach
★ kale	★ corn
★ broccoli	★ zucchini
★ collard greens	★ romaine lettuce
★ green peas	★ brussels sprouts

research suggests your body may absorb lutein from egg yolks more easily than from leafy greens. What's more, one study shows that eggs may not raise cholesterol and triglycerides as once thought. So consider enjoying an egg every now and again. You can also try other lutein and zeaxanthin sources, such as orange bell peppers, summer and winter squash, corn, broccoli, mustard greens, and kiwi fruit.

Wise way to counteract cataracts

You might not think of spinach and other leafy greens as "eye candy," but they contain real treats for your eyes. These "treats" — lutein and zeaxanthin — are amazing nutrients that may help you avoid cataracts, surgery, and even blindness.

This sounds too good to be true, but Harvard research suggests it really works. A 10-year study of over 35,000 women found that those who got the most lutein and zeaxanthin — about 6 milligrams — were 18 percent less likely to get cataracts than those who got the least. Scientists think these nutrients can help foil the process that helps cause cataracts.

Here's what happens. Your body regularly produces free radicals — unstable molecules that can cause cell damage. They're like gangs of thieves and vandals roaming your body. As if that weren't bad enough, hazards like ultraviolet light from the sun can make your eyes produce extra free radicals. Over time, these hoards of free radicals cause the lens of your eye to change in ways that lead to cataracts. But lutein and zeaxanthin can help prevent that. They're able to enter the lens of your eye and take on free radicals right where they live. And because lutein and zeaxanthin are antioxidants, they can render those free radicals harmless.

To get the most out of these nutrients, you should know two things.

- Your best sources of lutein include spinach, dandelion greens, kale, turnip greens, mustard greens, and collards.

- Your body can absorb more lutein and zeaxanthin if you eat these foods with a little fat. Fortunately, the Harvard researchers also found that vitamin E can help you avoid cataracts. So to get the most benefits, eat your lutein-rich foods with vitamin-E rich foods containing some healthy fats, like vegetable oils and almonds.

Foil a future heart attack

Heart attacks may seem to happen suddenly, but they're actually years in the making. Fortunately, the same lutein-rich foods that protect your eyes may also help defend your heart. According to a University of Southern California study, middle-age people who got the most lutein from their diets had the least narrowing of their arteries over 18 months — in fact, almost none at all. That's important because heart attacks happen when an artery can't deliver oxygen-rich blood to the heart muscle because it has narrowed to the point of being completely clogged.

Artery blockages may take years to form, but they start with some-thing called free radicals. Free radicals are unstable molecules that form when your body processes oxygen. Unless they're stopped by antioxidants, like lutein, these molecules can cause irreversible damage. Free radicals and antioxidants fight a war over your health every day, including frequent battles inside your arteries.

Unfortunately, each battle you lose may bring you closer to a heart attack and here's why. When free radicals attack your LDL choles-terol, they turn it into oxidized LDL. Oxidized LDL sticks to your artery walls and forms a lining of plaque. Each time more LDL is oxidized, more plaque can form. Over the years, that plaque builds up like gunk inside a drainpipe, and your arteries grow narrower and narrower until a blockage — and a heart attack — occur. But lutein can jump in and keep LDL from getting oxidized — lowering your risk of a future heart attack just a little bit more. So eat lutein-rich foods, like leafy greens, every day. You may be trimming your heart attack risk every time.

Magnesium

Balance blood sugar with a marvelous mineral

Your body needs magnesium to help your muscles and nerves work, keep your heart healthy, and boost your bones and immune system. If you're older than 55, you're likely low on magnesium. Some 90 percent of adults don't get enough of this important mineral, and seniors are the most at risk. Not only do older adults get less magnesium in their diets, their bodies absorb less from foods and excrete more in urine. Even worse, seniors are more likely to take drugs that interfere with magnesium absorption from foods. That adds up to a higher risk of deficiency. That's really bad news if you have diabetes.

Diabetes changes how your body uses energy from food. Since magnesium helps your body use carbohydrates and affects insulin levels, this mineral is important to help regulate your blood sugar. If you don't get enough magnesium, the enzymes involved in blood sugar metabolism may not function properly, making you resistant to insulin.

In fact, several studies have shown a connection between how much magnesium you get in your diet and how likely you are to develop diabetes. A summary of research on this subject found that people who get the most magnesium have a risk of developing type 2 diabetes that's 23 percent lower than people who get the least magnesium. Some experts suggest that people with type 2 diabetes take magnesium supplements to help control blood sugar. To find out if it's a good idea for you, ask your doctor.

Super sources of magnesium

★ spinach	★ turnip greens
★ halibut	★ collard greens
★ mollusks	★ pumpkin seeds
★ peanuts	★ sesame seeds
★ almonds	★ black beans

Pathway to lower blood pressure and a healthy heart

Magnesium, along with calcium and potassium, are important electrolytes that help regulate your blood pressure. Some experts think getting enough of these minerals is even more important than reducing salt intake in the battle against high blood pressure.

What's more, many scientists think too little magnesium in your body may be the missing link between simply having heart disease risk factors and actually developing heart disease. Not enough magnesium can cause a dangerous chain reaction within your cells and blood vessels that results in narrowed arteries, blood clots, and a buildup of cholesterol in your bloodstream. Because magnesium also works as a blood thinner, your levels of this mineral must be checked if you take certain drugs, like diuretics.

Here's a nutrient-rich eating plan that can help lower your blood pressure. It also raises your antioxidant intake to keep cholesterol under control and prevent heart disease. The DASH diet — Dietary Approaches to Stop Hypertension — focuses on delicious, healthy foods. It includes lots of fruits, vegetables, and legumes, many of them high in magnesium and other helpful minerals. The DASH diet aims to limit salt, saturated fats, and meat, while boosting your intake of monounsaturated fats — like olive oil — and whole grains. There's little evidence to show magnesium supplements will help your heart, so stick to this amazing diet that gives you plenty of the mighty mineral naturally.

Household Hint

Clean glassware with ease

You can do more with magnesium-loaded beans than just eat them. They're also handy cleaning helpers. Use them to scour the insides of slender glass vases. Fill the vase halfway with water and a bit of bleach. Then add a handful of dried beans or peas to the container. Swirl the mixture and let the beans scrub away the stains for you.

Cancel out colon cancer

When your tummy feels bad, you may reach for MOM — Milk of Magnesia, that is. It works as a laxative to make your bowels regular and as an antacid to soothe your stomach. The magnesium in MOM and in your food may also ward off colon cancer.

This deadly form of cancer, which is more common as people get older, may be linked to eating too much meat and not enough magnesium-rich fruits and vegetables, like green leafy vegetables, beans, and nuts. In fact, research shows that people who get more magnesium in their diets have a lower risk of developing colon cancer. The well-known Iowa Women's Health Study recorded what foods middle-age women ate most often and then followed their health for 17 years. Women who got the most magnesium — mostly from food but also from supplements — had the lowest risk of developing colon cancer.

Researchers can't explain the connection for sure, but they suggest magnesium lowers oxidative stress, or fights free radicals that can cause cell damage. Magnesium may also stop the growth of new — possibly cancerous — cells in the wall of the colon. Fiber in the same foods that have lots of magnesium may also provide protection.

Soothing bath boosts your magnesium

Most people don't get the recommended daily amount of magnesium — 420 milligrams (mg) for men and 320 mg for women. You can up your intake by eating magnesium-rich foods like greens, beans, nuts, and seeds. You can also get magnesium from supplements, but don't overdo it. Too much can cause diarrhea and abdominal cramps. Excess magnesium is especially dangerous if you have kidney problems, because your kidneys have to work hard to get rid of it.

Here's another way to raise your magnesium level naturally and safely — take a bath in Epsom salts, also known as magnesium sulfate. One study found that people who soaked in Epsom salts for just 12 minutes each day for a week enjoyed a boost in magnesium. Use about 2 1/2 cups of Epsom salts in your bathtub, and bathe two or three times a week. It's a great way to get more of this important mineral.

Mag-nificent way to better health

Magnesium in your diet is a jack of all trades — a true Renaissance mineral. It works hard to keep your bones, muscles, and nerves functioning as they should.

Put restlessness to rest. Magnesium may help battle a secret cause of fatigue and muscle spasms — a condition called restless legs syndrome (RLS). People with RLS feel an urge to move their feet or legs repeatedly, just when they're trying to rest or sleep. This can lead to lack of sleep and fatigue.

Not getting enough magnesium may be part of the problem because magnesium works with calcium to control how nerves tell muscles to contract. Without enough magnesium, your muscles get confused and can have spasms or cramps. One small study found that people with RLS who took magnesium supplements every evening had less trouble with leg movements during the night and slept better.

Bank on better bones. Most of the magnesium in your body is stored in your bones. It resides there along with calcium and phosphorous, keeping your bones strong. But if you develop osteoporosis, those bones can turn into something more like Swiss cheese, weakened from the missing minerals. Magnesium helps your bones hold on to calcium to maintain bone strength as you age. In fact, research shows getting too little magnesium may lead to thinning bones.

Hide out from headaches. You need enough magnesium in your body to prevent migraines if you're prone to these overpowering headaches. That's because a lack of this mineral causes a chain of events in your brain, which ends with constricted blood vessels and migraine pain. Magnesium may also stave off migraines related to menstruation.

Defend your hearing. Get enough magnesium — along with vitamin A, vitamin C, and vitamin E — and you may be able to fend off noise-related hearing loss. That's what researchers found when they tried giving various combinations of nutrients to guinea pigs, then checking to see how loud noises damaged their hearing. Magnesium alone didn't help much, but the nutrient combination worked.

Make plans to load up on the high-magnesium foods that can cure you. Start with an oat bran muffin or cooked oat bran for breakfast, fit in a peanut butter sandwich for lunch, then enjoy halibut, collard greens, and black beans for dinner. Top it off with a dessert that includes walnuts and almonds, and you're on your way to better health.

Mangosteen

Unusual fruit promises top defense

The newest superfruit — mangosteen — is not related to the mango, although both are tropical fruits that may be rare in your local grocery store. Mangosteens grow mostly in Southeast Asia, where people have long used the fruit to treat wounds, diarrhea, pain, and inflammation.

Xanthones — special plant chemicals in mangosteens — are what set this fruit apart, earning it the label of "superfruit." Experts are working to find out just how these phytochemicals may help you stay healthy.

■ They fight inflammation. Lab research in mice found the two most important xanthones in the outer fleshy hulls of mangosteens keep inflammation from getting out of control. They do this by acting like COX-2 inhibitors — pain-relieving drugs like Celebrex.

■ They battle bacteria and fungi. Ever heard of MRSA? That's a type of bacterium that has become resistant to the usual antibiotics doctors use to stop infections. Early research shows xanthones from mangosteen work with certain antibiotics to send MRSA packing — good news for seniors, athletes, or anyone at risk from this deadly invader.

■ They combat cancer. Xanthones are powerful antioxidants, similar to vitamins A and C. That means they patrol your body, mopping up the dangerous free radicals that may lead to some types of cancers. Xanthones from mangosteens also kill cancer cells in colon cancer and leukemia. They do this by causing the cancer cells to commit suicide.

Research on the health benefits of mangosteen is still in the early stages, in spite of sensational advertising from some mangosteen juice manufacturers. In fact, the Food and Drug Administration warned one company to stop making claims of medical effects from its products. But you can still eat mangosteen just as you do other healthy fruits and vegetables, knowing the natural goodness of this tropical wonder is just what your body needs to perform at its healthiest.

Household Hint

Best buys on mangosteens

Fresh mangosteens are expensive — about $45 per pound or $10 for one piece of fruit. That's why the most common form you'll find is bottled juice, often a mixture of whole crushed fruit with other types of juices. You'll see ads from companies that sell mangosteen juice through a network of distributors, like XanGo and Thai-Go. Some companies make amazing claims for their products, and the prices are equally high. If $30 to $40 for a 32-ounce bottle of fruit juice seems excessive, you may find a "deal" of $18 at a warehouse store.

A cheaper solution may be to buy the fruit canned. You can probably find a 20-ounce can of mangosteen packed in syrup for just a few dollars. Try your local Asian or Thai grocery or health-food store.

How to eat a mangosteen

This ugly little fruit looks like a small round eggplant wearing a jaunty green cap. Here's how you get at the tasty insides.

- When a mangosteen is fresh off the tree, you can squeeze it until the outer skin splits. If it's older and the skin has dried and hardened, you'll need a knife.

- Cut a shallow line around the fruit's equator. Carefully twist open the fruit.

- You'll see slippery white segments inside, which you can scoop out and enjoy.

- A seed is inside most segments. It's bitter, so don't eat it.

- Store the opened mangosteen in a plastic bag in the refrigerator to keep it from drying out.

Superfruit keeps you super fresh

The exotic mangosteen may be the newest player in the personal-care game. This "queen of fruits" has inspired natural perfumes, and it's being developed into products to keep your body clean, fresh, and looking great.

- Mangosteen juice may work as a mouthwash to treat bad breath. A study of 60 people with gum disease — one of the few bits of mangosteen research done on people so far — found using the mouthwash twice a day for two weeks improved their bad breath. You can buy mangosteen mouthwash online that's made in Thailand, and it may soon be more widely available.

- An extract of mangosteen stops bacteria from causing redness and inflammation when you have acne. So if skin breakouts are a problem, mangosteen may be just the ticket to help keep it under control and avoid scars.

- The huge amount of antioxidants in mangosteen made researchers consider how it could keep your skin looking young. One study found a cream with mangosteen, tea, and pomegranate extracts worked wonders in repairing sun damage to the skin of women who used it.

Who needs everyday botanicals like oatmeal and aloe when mangosteen can make you look and feel like a queen?

Nuts

Say 'nuts' to a heart attack

You may have heard almonds are the one nut that's good for your heart, but that's not entirely true. You'll find at least five other delicious nuts that may also help you avoid a heart attack.

Pistachios. People who ate 3 ounces of pistachios a day lowered their "bad" LDL cholesterol by more than 11 percent in a single month, a small Penn State University study reports. As if that weren't enough, as little as 1 1/2 ounces of pistachios a day helped reduce oxidized LDL cholesterol — the kind most likely to lead to plaque, clogged arteries, and heart attacks. The scientists behind the study think the pistachio's lutein, a phytochemical, and gamma tocopherol, a kind of vitamin E, may help prevent LDL from becoming oxidized.

Macadamias. Along with the oxidation of LDL cholesterol, inflammation in your arteries is also a key ingredient for a future heart attack.

But a study of 17 men with high cholesterol found that those who added 1 1/2 ounces, about a small handful, of macadamia nuts to their diets reduced signs of inflammation and oxidation in their arteries.

Walnuts. Volunteers who ate about a half ounce of walnuts every day for two months had 17 percent lower triglycerides and 9 percent higher "good" HDL cholesterol than people who didn't, a study from Iran's Shiraz University found.

Hazelnuts. In just two months, 15 men with high cholesterol lowered their triglycerides by 30 percent and increased their HDL cholesterol by 12 percent, say scientists from Turkey's Hacettepe University. They also reduced several other heart attack risk factors. Their secret? A low-fat, low-cholesterol, high-carbohydrate diet that included about 1 1/2 ounces of hazelnuts, or filberts, every day.

Peanuts. Although technically a legume and not a nut, these tasty morsels are very heart friendly. Men who ate about a half cup of peanuts every day lowered their total triglycerides by 20 percent in just eight weeks. They also cut their total cholesterol, reports a small study from Ghana's Food Research Institute.

Of course, none of these studies was large enough to be indisputable proof, and some of them were funded by organizations such as the California Pistachio Commission or the Hazelnut Promotion group. That's why more research is needed. But don't think this means these studies can't be right. In fact, you'll find several reasons why nuts may be just the food you need for a healthier heart.

■ Nuts contain compounds called phytosterols. These compounds keep your intestines from absorbing cholesterol to send to your bloodstream. What's more, the fiber, monounsaturated fats, and polyunsaturated fats in nuts also help keep your cholesterol down.

■ The copper in nuts can help protect your heart from the effects of stress and may help prevent an enlarged heart.

- Nuts contain arginine, an amino acid that helps prevent LDL oxidation in your arteries.

- Nuts give you minerals that help control blood pressure.

But how you include nuts in your diet may well determine whether they help you or not. Adding nuts on top of a diet that's already high in fat may lead to weight gain, which hurts your heart. Use nuts to replace less-healthy foods in your diet, such as French fries, candy bars, meats, and other foods high in saturated fats or empty calories. A handful or two of nuts a day could make all the difference.

Household Hint

Discover almond milk and almond butter

Crunchy almonds are delicious, but you haven't discovered true almond joy until you've tried almond butter and almond milk. Almond butter is just like peanut butter — but made with almonds. You'll pay a high price for this delicious food in the store, so make your own at home. You'll need 3/4 cup of ground, blanched almonds, a pinch of salt, and 2 tablespoons of canola oil. Place the ground almonds and salt in your blender or food processor with one tablespoon of oil. Mix, add the second tablespoon of oil, and then blend until smooth.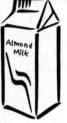

Almond milk is an almond-flavored substitute for milk that you may find in the natural foods section of your super-market. Use it in place of milk or creamer when making coffee or hot chocolate. If you can't tolerate milk, substitute almond milk for the real thing. You can also mix almond milk with yogurt and frozen fruit for a tantalizing smoothie.

Nutty way to fight diabetes

Keeping your blood sugar down can be tough whether you're worried about getting diabetes or you already have it. But now you have a crunchy ally to help you fend off after dinner spikes in blood sugar and lower your risk of diabetes — nuts. According to a small University of Toronto study, people made less insulin each day when they snacked on almonds instead of a whole-wheat muffin. That's important because rising insulin production can be a sign you're developing insulin resistance and possibly diabetes.

Normally, your body can lower its blood sugar by transporting that sugar into your liver and muscle cells. But just as you need a guest pass to get into your favorite warehouse club, blood sugar needs insulin to get into cells. Unfortunately, in some people, those cells lose their ability to accept blood sugar. When that happens, your body panics and makes more insulin to overcome this "insulin resistance." This torrent of insulin gets blood sugar into your cells, but after awhile, your insulin-making cells begin to wear out from overwork. Then insulin starts tapering off and your blood sugar begins to rise. Fortunately, nuts can help both your insulin and blood sugar levels.

Eating 3 ounces of almonds with white bread reduced the total Glycemic Index (GI) — or how fast blood sugar rises after eating a food — of the bread by half, report University of Toronto scientists. The scientists think eating almonds with a meal blunts the post-meal blood sugar rise, but eating almonds as a snack throughout the day may rein in insulin production all day long.

Although both Canadian studies used almonds, other studies suggest even peanuts will do. A small Arizona State University study found that peanuts can help hold down the blood sugar spikes that follow meals with a high GI. What's more, women who ate a handful of nuts five or more times a week were 27 percent less likely to develop diabetes than women who avoided eating nuts, according to the famous Nurses' Health Study.

The secret behind this nutty success may be the healthy monounsaturated fats in nuts, but your secret to success is making sure you eat nuts the right way. Use nuts in place of high carbohydrate foods — especially the ones high in fat. Not only will you replace unhealthy fats with good fats, you'll also lower the GI of your meals. And that could mean diabetes may not be such a tough nut to crack after all.

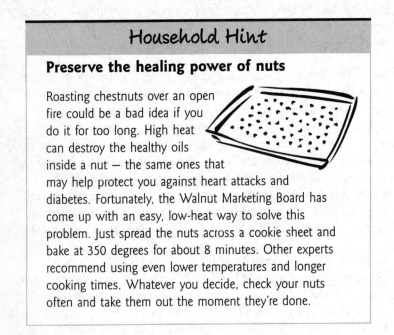

Household Hint

Preserve the healing power of nuts

Roasting chestnuts over an open fire could be a bad idea if you do it for too long. High heat can destroy the healthy oils inside a nut — the same ones that may help protect you against heart attacks and diabetes. Fortunately, the Walnut Marketing Board has come up with an easy, low-heat way to solve this problem. Just spread the nuts across a cookie sheet and bake at 350 degrees for about 8 minutes. Other experts recommend using even lower temperatures and longer cooking times. Whatever you decide, check your nuts often and take them out the moment they're done.

The real truth about nuts and weight

You might think nuts are worse than cake when it comes to piling on the pounds, but that's just a tired old myth. In fact, nuts might even help keep you from gaining weight.

People who eat nuts at least twice a week are less likely to put on pounds than people who never eat nuts, reports a study from Spain's University of Navarra. In fact, nut lovers had 30 percent lower odds of gaining 11 pounds or more during the 28-month study. What's more, the people who ate nuts more frequently gained the least weight.

Believe it or not, the high protein and fat in nuts may help your body resist weight gain. Healthy, unsaturated fats may team up with protein to rev up your calorie-burning powers. Meanwhile, the fiber in nuts may also help you absorb less fat. But this doesn't mean you can fill up on burgers, shakes, fries, and cake. Instead, include nuts in a diet full of low-fat, high-fiber favorites to get the most bang for your buck.

Oatmeal

Basic breakfast guards your heart

The heart-healthy labels on oatmeal boxes aren't just for looks. This simple hot cereal has a proven record protecting you from heart disease.

Controls cholesterol. Chow down on this cholesterol sponge. A meta-analysis of eight studies showed oats lowered both total and "bad" LDL cholesterol. Most importantly, LDL dropped an average of 5 percent. It may not sound like much, but even this small change could cut your risk of heart disease 5 to 15 percent. That's because every 1 percent drop in your LDL cholesterol results in 1 to 3 percent less chance of developing heart disease.

The soluble fiber in oats, called beta glucan, is much better at lowering cholesterol than the insoluble fiber in other grains, like wheat. You need to eat about 15 grams of oat fiber daily to see significant changes in your cholesterol level, but you don't have to eat it all as oatmeal. Look for breads made with oat flour, and use it to bake your own goods. Read labels and choose prepackaged oat products with the most fiber per serving.

Defends your arteries. Some LDL cholesterol is worse than others. Small, densely packed LDL particles are more likely to oxidize than large, less dense LDL, a process that leads to closed up arteries. New evidence suggests oats are especially good at cutting down the number of small, dense LDL particles. In a group of overweight men, half ate oat bran cereals, and half ate whole wheat cereals. Here's what happened.

	Small-density LDL	Large-density LDL	Total LDL
Oat group	dropped 16%	increased 13%	dropped 5%
Wheat group	increased 59%	dropped 15%	increased 14%

Remember, the goal is to lower your levels of small-density and total LDL as much as possible. Oats beat wheat hands down. Consider swapping that bowl of Wheaties for slow-cooked oatmeal.

Beats high blood pressure. Having high blood pressure is a major risk factor for heart disease, but oats can knock it down a notch. Eating foods made with oat fiber lowered both systolic and diastolic blood pressure in obese people. High blood pressure may be linked to insulin problems. Foods like oats help kill two birds with one stone, balancing insulin levels and keeping blood pressure in line. Experts say obese people may benefit most from oats, because they are more likely to have insulin problems.

Prevents blocked blood vessels. Humble oats have a secret weapon — antioxidants known as avenanthramides (AVs). When blood vessels get damaged, immune cells rush to the area to repair them. Then, smooth muscle grows inside the vessels, where it doesn't belong, and ultimately artery-clogging plaques start to form. Lab tests show AVs put the brakes on this process by stopping immune cells from attaching to blood vessels and preventing the overgrowth of smooth muscle.

Heads off heart disease. Oats pack the powerful punch of whole grains, too. Whole grains contain a network of nutrients, including fiber, vitamins, minerals, and phytochemicals, that work together to fight heart disease. In fact, eating three or more servings of whole grains, like oats, daily is linked to a lower risk of heart disease, not to mention diabetes and obesity — two more risk factors in its development.

Dynamic duo powers up protection

Get more heart-helping power from your morning oatmeal by drinking a glass of orange juice. The antioxidants in oats and the juice's vitamin C work together to keep LDL cholesterol from oxidizing. OJ and oatmeal each prevent this process on their own, but they're even more effective when taken together.

Slimming oats help you watch your waistline

Some of the healthiest foods are actually the cheapest. A breakfast of oatmeal costs less than 50 cents, but it can help you lose weight and lower your cholesterol.

Eating a fiber-rich diet with food like oats makes you less likely to become obese. People who eat plenty of fiber:

■ feel less hungry between meals.

■ fill up faster during meals, so they eat less.

■ eat fewer total calories throughout the day.

High-fiber eaters also tend to be leaner. Women who upped their fiber intake over the course of 12 years were half as likely to gain 55 pounds or more than women who ate less fiber over time. In fact, ramping up your fiber intake by 14 grams a day can help you lose weight — 4 pounds over four months, on average — without changing your lifestyle.

Beta glucan, the same soluble oat fiber that puts a lid on your cholesterol, dissolves in liquid and forms a gel around food in your gut. This slows down the passage of food through your digestive tract, so you feel full longer. It may also prevent your body from absorbing unhealthy fats in food, thereby cutting the calories you get. Dress it up with fresh blueberries or sliced strawberries or peaches for a fruity, high-fiber breakfast that keeps your energy up throughout a busy morning.

Oats are whole grains, too, and eating three or more servings of whole grains daily can help you maintain your weight and avoid putting on pounds over the years. Plus, oatmeal takes up a lot of space in your belly but has few calories. And studies show it can make you feel fuller than other whole-grain cereals or breads with the same amount of calories.

Still, even the most fiber-filled meal won't stop weight gain if it's also packed with sugar and fat. Avoid instant oatmeal loaded with added sugar. Newer "weight control" oatmeals boast added protein and extra fiber, giving you the belly-busting benefits of both nutrients in your morning meal. Research suggests breakfasts high in protein but low in saturated fat can help you eat less the rest of the day.

Balance blood sugar with a breakfast basic

Oats could be your ticket to getting control of diabetes. Beta glucan, the soluble fiber in oats, seems to keep a lid on insulin and blood sugar spikes after meals.

Once in your stomach, it becomes a gel which slows the movement of food through your digestive system. It also slows the digestion of carbohydrates, so their sugars don't hit your bloodstream all at once. Instead, you get a gradual rise in blood sugar and insulin — a real boon for people with diabetes trying to keep tight control of their blood sugar.

What's more, soluble fiber ferments once it reaches your colon. This process releases fatty acids that may regulate how your liver responds to blood sugar levels. Eating foods full of beta glucan may improve how your body handles glucose in the long-term.

You need at least 4 grams of beta glucan in a meal to get these benefits. The more processed the oats, the less beta glucan they likely contain, since processing can break down this fiber. Choose steel-cut oats over instant, and don't count on oatmeal cookies to suddenly become good for you. Baking seems to break down beta glucan, too.

Ease IBS symptoms with oats

Does your digestive system benefit more from savory breads and cereals or from scrumptious fruits and vegetables? If you suffer from IBS, the insoluble fiber in cold cereals, whole grains, and wheat products can make your symptoms worse. Gentler sources of soluble fiber — the kind found in oats, beans, vegetables, and fruits — can help.

Besides soaking up LDL cholesterol and controlling blood sugar, soluble oat fiber aids in digestion, too. A review of 17 studies found that increasing soluble fiber improved overall IBS symptoms. Bumping up insoluble fiber, however, did not. In some cases, it even worsened IBS symptoms.

If you suffer constipation along with IBS, aim to get between 12 and 30 grams of soluble fiber daily from oats, lentils, fruits, and other foods. Increase your fiber slowly to avoid bloating and gas, and drink plenty of fluids to help your body process the extra bulk. Be careful about boosting your fiber intake if diarrhea is your main IBS symptom, since extra fiber may worsen it.

Enjoy clearer, younger-looking skin

Oats do more than ease poison ivy itch. They can also improve rosacea symptoms, make you look younger, and help wounds heal faster.

Put an end to itching. The same compounds that help oats fight heart disease may also soothe itchy skin. Avenanthramides (AVs), the antioxidants found only in oats, soothed skin inflammation and eased itching in a study on sensitive skin — further proof that oatmeal baths really do soothe itchy rashes and bug bites.

Rise above rosacea. These same properties make oatmeal an excellent treatment for rosacea. Colloidal oatmeal, the powder made from grinding whole oat grains, is a natural skin protectant.

- Proteins and polysaccharides form a protective shield and buffer skin against everyday assault from other compounds.

- Its natural oils keep skin from drying out.

- Saponins gently absorb dirt and oil, while other oat compounds break down pollutants.

Colloidal oatmeal is also a powerful anti-inflammatory. It cuts the formation of prostaglandins, inflammation-causing compounds, up to 85 percent, results similar to what you'd get with a topical anti-inflammatory medicine. Add them together, and oatmeal packs real promise in treating rosacea.

Erase lines and wrinkles. Oats may contain a miracle anti-aging substance that cosmetics only dream of. Applying a special rub made from beta glucan, the soluble fiber in oats, for eight weeks made skin look smoother and reduced wrinkles and fine lines. Beta glucan penetrated skin and promoted the buildup of collagen, which helps tighten skin and reduce the look of fine lines and wrinkles.

Heal wounds faster. Rubs containing beta glucan also seem to speed wound-healing, too, especially burns, shallow scratches, and laser treatments. Beta glucan:

- increases the number of immune system helpers in the hurt area.

- prompts your body to build new collagen, a building block of skin.

- promotes the growth of new skin layers to cover wounds.

- makes healed skin stronger and more flexible.

You can make your own oat baths, creams, and masks at home. Finely grind quick or old-fashioned oats in a food processor, then slowly sprinkle it under fast-running bath water for a colloidal oatmeal bath. For rubs and masks, mix your ground oatmeal or store-bought oat flour with just enough water to get the right consistency.

New hope for celiac disease

People suffering from celiac disease, an autoimmune disorder, are stuck with strict and sometimes boring diets. Oats may change that. Gluten, a protein found in foods, triggers an immune reaction in people with celiac. Their immune system attacks their small intestine, destroying part of it over time. This, in turn, can lead to malnutrition, diarrhea, anemia, and osteoporosis.

That's why it's crucial to avoid foods containing gluten if you have this condition. Wheat, rye, and barley, the main grains used in bread and baked goods, have lots of gluten. Oats, however, do not, and new studies show most people with celiac can safely eat them.

Oats can add variety to an otherwise bland celiac diet as well as boost its nutritional value. The catch — you can eat only pure oats, and no more than a half to three-quarters cup a day. Pure oats are grown and processed under controlled conditions to prevent contamination by wheat and other gluten-containing grains. They're already available in Canada. Look for them soon in the United States with the label "gluten-free."

Stop eating oats if your celiac symptoms return or worsen. A small percentage of people with the disease can't tolerate oats, either.

Low-Fat Oatmeal Cookies

Ingredients

3/4 cup sugar

2 Tbsp margarine

1/4 cup egg substitute

1/4 cup applesauce

2 Tbsp 1% milk

1 cup all-purpose flour

1/4 tsp baking soda

1/2 tsp ground cinnamon

1 cup rolled oats

Instructions

1. Preheat oven to 350°F, and lightly grease cookie sheets.

2. In a large bowl, use an electric mixer on medium speed to mix sugar and margarine. Mix until well blended, about 3 minutes.

3. Slowly add egg substitute. Mix on medium speed 1 minute. Gradually add applesauce and milk; mix on medium speed 1 minute. Scrape sides of bowl.

4. In another bowl, combine flour, baking soda, and cinnamon. Slowly add to applesauce mixture; mix on low speed until blended, about 2 minutes. Add oats and blend 30 seconds on low speed. Scrape sides of bowl.

5. Drop by teaspoonfuls onto cookie sheet, about 2 inches apart.

6. Bake until lightly browned, about 13 to 15 minutes. Remove from baking sheet while still warm. Cool on wire rack.

Serving size: 2 cookies

(Serves 8)

Nutrition Summary by Serving

206.1 Calories (35.5 calories from fat, 17.24 percent of total); 3.9 g Fats; 4.4 g Protein; 38.8 g Carbohydrates; 0.3 mg Cholesterol; 1.6 g Fiber; 94.1 mg Sodium

Olive oil

Change your oil for a healthier heart

Switch from spreading butter on your bread to dipping it in olive oil, and you'll be trading unhealthy saturated fats for healthier mono-unsaturated fatty acids (MUFAs). These so-called "healthy fats" are a big part of the Mediterranean diet — the traditional way of eating in countries that border the Mediterranean Sea, like Greece and Italy. Compared to a common Western diet, the Mediterranean diet includes lots of fruits and vegetables, whole grains and cereals, nuts and seeds, beans, and MUFAs, like olive oil. Dairy, red meat, poultry, and other sources of saturated fat are limited.

The Mediterranean Diet is not only tasty, it's great for your heart. The closer you stick to eating Mediterranean style, the lower your risk of dying from heart disease. You can credit olive oil's heart-healthy MUFAs and antioxidant polyphenols. Here's how they help.

- Raise your "good" HDL cholesterol and lower triglycerides. One study found that olive oil containing the most polyphenols, or natural antioxidants, improved the cholesterol levels of men who ate about one tablespoon of olive oil every day for three weeks. Less-refined oil, like virgin olive oil, contains more polyphenols, which means more health benefits.

- Bring down high blood pressure. Researchers found that people on a diet high in monounsaturated fats, like olive oil, enjoyed lower blood pressure than those on a high-carbohydrate diet.

- Clear away blood clots. The high content of phenolic compounds in virgin olive oil primes your body to prevent blood clots. This keeps your blood flowing more smoothly and lowers your risk of a heart attack or stroke.

- Protect your arteries. Researchers found that people who eat more olive oil have less thickening of their carotid arteries, a measure of atherosclerosis. That translates into less risk of hardening of the arteries and heart disease.

A traditional Mediterranean diet may also include a moderate amount of red wine. Experts found when you drink it with a meal that contains olive oil, the combination may lower your blood pressure and keep your blood flowing smoothly.

Oil your joints for soothing relief

Ever noticed that bitter taste in extra virgin olive oil? It's what makes good-quality olive oil the pantry favorite that's packed with a pain-fighting nutrient. You know about pain if you suffer from osteoarthritis (OA), a degenerative disease that makes your joints swell and ache. OA happens when the cartilage that normally cushions your joints begins to break down, causing inflammation and wear to your bones.

Nearly half of all people in the United States can expect to develop knee arthritis. You can try nonsteroidal anti-inflammatory drugs (NSAIDs), like aspirin or ibuprofen, for the swelling and pain, but some experts say they don't work well over time. People who use NSAIDs may still have pain — plus, they can develop serious side effects.

Instead, relieve your arthritic joints by switching to the salad oil with nutrients that work like Motrin to fight inflammation. Olive oil gets its pain-relieving power from an enzyme called oleocanthal. This bitter-tasting enzyme works a lot like ibuprofen and other anti-inflammatory drugs. Experts say you should aim for about 4 tablespoons of freshly pressed extra-virgin olive oil every day for the best results. That's about 476 calories, so you'll need to substitute this healthy fat for unhealthy fats in your diet.

Not surprisingly, olive oil is not just for salads. You can use it for cooking, too. Extra-virgin olive oil is great for dipping bread or adding a rich taste to pastas. You can also sauté and grill with it, but the higher the heat, the more you risk losing the oil's unique flavor.

Choose the right product for the job

Don't pick an olive oil based on price. Instead, consider these factors when you shop, and you'll bring home the best-tasting and most nutritious oil.

- **High quality.** Pick virgin or extra-virgin olive oil, which has the most antioxidant polyphenols. That's important to protect your heart and to reduce the formation of dangerous acrylamide compounds. These compounds form when you cook starchy foods at high heat, like frying. One study found you can safely fry potatoes using virgin olive oil with a high-phenol content.

- **Taste.** Avoid pomace oil, which is the cheapest, lowest-quality variety. It's made from the paste that's left after other types of oil have been extracted. Don't buy it to save money because it tastes horrible. In fact, if you think you don't like the taste of olive oil, you may have been trying pomace oil.

- **Color.** Oils can range from yellow to green, but color variation may be due to several factors. Green oil may be from green, barely ripe olives, giving it a good taste. Or it could be from leaves falling in the processor. Yellow oil may be from olives picked late in the season — or it may have oxidized from light exposure, which means fewer nutrients.

- **Packaging.** Look for oil in a dark glass bottle that prevents exposure to ultraviolet light. In that case, you won't be able to see the oil's color.

Look great for less with olive oil

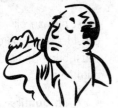

Replace costly products for your hair and skin with homemade blends made with olive oil. The all-natural goodness of this old-world oil can also help you keep unnecessary chemicals out of your house.

Condition your hair naturally. Mix together an egg yolk with 3 teaspoons each olive oil, honey, and lemon juice. Work through your hair and leave on for 15 minutes, then rinse and shampoo. Your hair will be soft, shiny, and moisturized.

Scrub your feet smooth. Combine 2 teaspoons olive oil, 3 tablespoons used coffee grounds, and 1 tablespoon each flour and heavy cream. Add a dash of cornmeal and several drops of your favorite scented oil and mix. Scrub the rough, dry parts of your feet, then rinse and pat dry. Dab on a touch of olive oil as a moisturizer.

Pamper your face. Use olive oil as a lubricant for close shaving or an eye makeup remover. You'll save money and make space on your bathroom counter.

Arm your colon with liquid gold

Add some olive oil to your daily diet, and you may be cutting down on your risk for colon cancer, the third most common cancer in men and women. Cancer of the colon, or large intestine, is less common in Mediterranean countries than in Northern Europe. Experts think olive oil in the Mediterranean diet may provide protection. Virgin and extra-virgin olive oil, the kinds with the least amount of processing, contain the most phenols. These natural antioxidants have anti-inflamma-tory powers, so researchers wondered how they might affect cancer cells.

In a lab study, phenols from olive oil stopped colon cancer cells from developing, and it blocked damage to cell DNA. When cancer cells are stopped from growing, they can't develop into tumors and spread. Monounsaturated fats in olive oil also lower the level of deoxycholic acid in your colon, a bile acid that encourages tumors to grow.

Olive oil may protect you from colon cancer in another way. Use it to cook meat and other protein-rich food, and it seems to reduce the amount of dangerous heterocyclic amines that are produced during cooking, especially frying. Researchers found that people who used olive oil to fry foods had a lower risk of developing colon cancer than people who used other fats, like peanut oil or butter.

Say goodbye to stomach pain

New research shows olive oil battles the type of bacteria that cause stomach ulcers and gastric, or stomach, cancer. Experts believe most stomach ulcers are caused by the bacterium *Helicobacter pylori (H. pylori)*, which burrows into your stomach lining and secretes toxins that cause inflammation and damage to the lining. *H. pylori* is also thought to be a cause of stomach cancer. Doctors prescribe antibiotics to kill *H. pylori*, but some strains are becoming resistant to the most commonly used antibiotics. That's why experts looked for another way to keep *H. pylori* at bay.

New research shows the phenolic compounds in virgin olive oil are natural bacteria killers. They work against several strains of *H. pylori*, including some of the antibiotic-resistant types. Even better, these phenolic compounds seem to keep working in strong stomach acid, so olive oil can fight *H. pylori* where it lurks.

So far, experts have tested olive oil in the lab rather than on people, so they don't know exactly how much olive oil you need to eat to win the battle against ulcers and stomach cancer. But since virgin olive oil contains a high concentration of phenolic compounds, it gives stronger protection than tea, wine, or other plant sources of these helpful, natural chemicals.

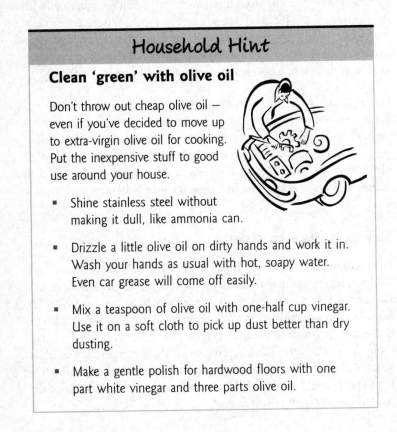

Household Hint

Clean 'green' with olive oil

Don't throw out cheap olive oil — even if you've decided to move up to extra-virgin olive oil for cooking. Put the inexpensive stuff to good use around your house.

- Shine stainless steel without making it dull, like ammonia can.

- Drizzle a little olive oil on dirty hands and work it in. Wash your hands as usual with hot, soapy water. Even car grease will come off easily.

- Mix a teaspoon of olive oil with one-half cup vinegar. Use it on a soft cloth to pick up dust better than dry dusting.

- Make a gentle polish for hardwood floors with one part white vinegar and three parts olive oil.

Stop aging in its tracks

Eating a Mediterranean diet, with lots of olive oil, fruits and vegetables, nuts and seeds, and breads and cereals, may help more than just your heart. It may also help you control diabetes, keep your weight in check, and stave off memory loss to help you stay young.

Keep diabetes under control. Researchers studied postmenopausal women with type 2 diabetes to see how following a Mediterranean diet and lifestyle could help. They found that women who changed their eating habits — and made other changes like exercising and lowering stress — were healthier after a year. They took in fewer calories from saturated fat and had greater improvements in heart disease risk factors. Another study found a Mediterranean diet may even help you sidestep developing type 2 diabetes in the first place.

Lose weight and keep it off. Unlike some weight loss plans that limit what you can eat, the Mediterranean diet includes a variety of tasty foods. That may make it easier to stick with in the long run. One study found that a moderate-fat diet, like Mediterranean-style eating, worked better for weight loss than a low-fat diet. Another study found a Mediterranean diet worked nearly as well as a low-carbohydrate diet, helping people lose an average of about 10 pounds over two years.

Head off Alzheimer's disease. Following a Mediterranean diet could lower your risk of developing this memory-stealing disease. The eating plan also may help people with Alzheimer's disease (AD) live longer. Researchers found that people with AD who followed a Mediterranean diet lived about four years longer than people who ate a typical Western diet.

Omega-3

Eat your way to lower blood pressure

High blood pressure makes your heart work harder and puts you at greater risk for heart disease and stroke. Luckily, you don't have to work too hard to bring your blood pressure down. Just get more omega-3 fatty acids into your diet.

Studies show that dietary supplements of omega-3 fatty acids lower blood pressure in people with high or normal blood pressure. Just 3 grams of eicosapentaenoic acid (EPA) and docosahexaenoic acid (DHA) — the omega-3 fatty acids found in fish — can lower systolic blood pressure by 5 millimeters of mercury (mm Hg) and diastolic blood pressure by 3 mm Hg.

But you don't need supplements to reap the benefit of omega-3. A recent study of more than 4,000 middle-aged people from China, Japan, the United Kingdom, and the United States found that eating foods rich in omega-3 can also help. Researchers aren't sure how omega-3 lowers blood pressure, but it may help relax and dilate your blood vessels by boosting nitric oxide production in the thin layer of cells that line blood vessels.

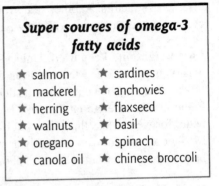

Super sources of omega-3 fatty acids

- ★ salmon
- ★ mackerel
- ★ herring
- ★ walnuts
- ★ oregano
- ★ canola oil
- ★ sardines
- ★ anchovies
- ★ flaxseed
- ★ basil
- ★ spinach
- ★ chinese broccoli

Besides fatty fish like salmon, mackerel, and sardines, other sources of omega-3 include canola oil, flaxseeds, and walnuts. These foods provide a type of omega-3 fatty acid called alpha-linolenic acid (ALA), which your body converts to DHA and EPA. A 1-percent increase in your blood levels of ALA means a 5 mm Hg drop in blood pressure. While omega-3's effects on blood pressure may be modest, every bit helps. Make omega-3-rich foods part of a healthy diet that includes limiting salt, alcohol, and saturated fat and getting enough potassium and calcium.

Fish oil keeps cholesterol under control

Tired of the ups and downs of watching your cholesterol? When you add more omega-3 fatty acids to your diet, you get much better ups and downs — good HDL cholesterol levels go up while dangerous triglyceride levels go down.

High-density lipoprotein (HDL) cholesterol whisks cholesterol to your liver and out of your body instead of carrying it to your artery walls. While you want to lower other types of cholesterol, you actually want to raise HDL levels to protect your heart and arteries. Triglycerides, on the other hand, cause nothing but trouble. These fats in the blood increase your risk of heart disease. By raising one and lowering the other, omega-3 fatty acids work doubly hard to help your heart.

Fatty fish, like wild salmon, halibut, and tuna, are your best source of omega-3 fatty acids, including eicosapentaeonic acid (EPA) and docosahexaenoic acid (DHA). If you don't like seafood, you can also take fish oil capsules. Aim for 3 grams of EPA and DHA. Talk to your doctor if you're taking blood thinners, like warfarin, before trying fish oil supplements.

Another option is flaxseed, which provides another type of omega-3 fatty acid called alpha-linolenic acid. Just one to three tablespoons of ground flaxseed daily should do the trick.

'Berry' good way to get omega-3

You don't need to eat fish to boost your intake of omega-3 fatty acids. In fact, you can find omega-3 in some surprising places — like blueberries. A recent Norwegian study found that blueberries contain a similar amount of alpha-linolenic acid as some wild green vegetables known for being rich in ALA.

Bone up on omega-3 to avoid osteoporosis

You already know how important calcium is when it comes to strong bones. But omega-3 fatty acids may also play a key role in bone health. A recent Penn State study found that plant sources of omega-3 could help prevent bone loss.

For more information on omega-3 fatty acids, see the Fish and Flaxseed chapters.

In the 23-person study, researchers controlled everything the people ate. They compared a standard American diet with those high in alpha-linolenic acid (ALA), an omega-3 fatty acid, and linoleic acid (LA), a type of omega-6 fatty acid.

The ALA diet led to a significant decrease in blood levels of N-telopeptides, a marker of bone loss. Meanwhile, markers of bone formation remained unchanged. In other words, you're still building bones, but they're not breaking down as much. That's a good recipe for avoiding osteoporosis.

Walnuts, which provide both ALA and LA, made up a large part of the diet. Besides snacking on walnuts, people in the study ate foods like walnut granola, honey walnut butter, and walnut pesto. Flaxseed oil also boosted ALA levels.

The key is the ratio of omega-6 to omega-3 in your diet. By eating more walnuts and flaxseed, you can add ALA while lowering the ratio — and raising your defense against osteoporosis.

Soothe psoriasis with fish oil

Like a creepy villain, psoriasis can make your skin crawl. With this chronic condition, you have dry, scaly, itchy, irritated patches of skin. You also have some hope, in the form of omega-3 fatty acids. Several studies show that fish oil supplements can help improve symptoms of psoriasis. Omega-3 probably helps because of its anti-inflammatory powers.

Adding support to that theory is the fact that high levels of arachidonic acid, a type of omega-6 fatty acid that promotes inflammation, are found in psoriatic skin lesions. Omega-3 fatty acids can counteract omega-6 to keep inflammation under control.

Getting more omega-3 into your diet, through either food or supplements, could help save your skin.

Onions & leeks

Nip a heart attack in the bud

You wouldn't use onions to protect your outdoor plumbing during a cold snap, but they may be a great way to protect your inner plumbing — the vital arteries that lead to your heart. Here's how the onion may defend your arteries and help you avoid a heart attack.

Onions are loaded with all kinds of health-giving compounds. One of them, quercetin, is already famous because it shows promise against allergy symptoms and high blood pressure. But scientists from England's Institute of Food Research think quercetin might also help fight one of the earliest building blocks for a heart attack — inflammation in your arteries.

The English scientists decided to put quercetin to the test. But since they wanted to simulate conditions that happen in the body, they couldn't test quercetin alone and here's why. When you digest onions, your body interacts with quercetin to produce new compounds called metabolites. What reaches your intestines isn't onion or quercetin — but rather the metabolites. It's these compounds that make their way into your bloodstream. Because the scientists knew this, they tested both quercetin and the metabolites on cells from the inner linings of arteries. They discovered that cells exposed to either quercetin or the metabolites limited the activity of key molecules that help cause inflammation. If onions can help prevent this inflammation, they may help prevent a heart attack, too.

Inflammation in your artery walls may begin long before a heart attack happens, but that doesn't make it any less dangerous. That's because inflammation is a key ingredient for creating plaque along the inner lining of your arteries. The more inflammation and plaque you have, the narrower your arteries become. In other words, it's like throwing rocks in a stream. If you keep doing it long enough, you'll eventually clog the stream. When a clog keeps oxygen-rich blood from getting to your heart, it triggers a heart attack.

Every time you prevent inflammation in your arteries, you may be preventing plaque, too. Less plaque means less chance you'll clog an artery and have a heart attack. That's a good reason to start enjoying more onions every day. You can defend your heart by adding onions to stir-fries, stews, and soups.

Delicious way to lower cancer risk

Add more onions and garlic to your marinades and you might lower your risk of cancer. Scientists from Germany's Hohenheim University marinated meats with several marinades, cooked them, and then tested them for cancer-causing compounds. The more onions and garlic the scientists put in the marinade, the fewer cancer-causing compounds formed in the meat. The next time you get ready to grill or fry beef, whip up an oil-based marinade with plenty of onions and garlic. Not only will it taste delicious, it may help keep you from getting cancer, too.

Dodge a very deadly cancer

Eating onions may help you avoid one of the deadliest cancers you can get — pancreatic cancer. Fewer than 4 percent of people diagnosed with cancer of the pancreas are alive five years later. But, like all cancers, this cancer can only pose a threat if it gets the chance to develop in your body. Fortunately, you can take steps to avoid this — and eating onions is a great way to start.

According to scientists from the University of California, San Francisco, people who eat the most onions and garlic are 54 percent less likely to get pancreatic cancer than those who eat the least. Experts suspect this happens because every onion has its own SWAT team of amazing nutrients. These powerful protectors may help your body fight off changes that can lead to pancreatic cancer.

But eating more onions doesn't just cut your risk of pancreatic cancer. A European study found that one to six servings of onions a week also cuts your risk of colorectal cancer, cancer of the larynx, and ovarian cancer. People who eat seven or more servings a week have a lower risk of mouth cancer and cancer of the esophagus.

One of the possible causes of many cancers is free radicals. Free radicals are unstable molecules produced every time you breathe. Unless they're stopped by antioxidants, they can damage your cells. Onions contain antioxidants and sulfur compounds to help neutralize free radicals. That makes it harder for cancer to get started and easier for you to stay healthy.

Super strategy for a healthy prostate

Everybody wants more get-up-and-go, but nobody wants to get up and go to the bathroom all night. Unfortunately, this problem is very common for men who develop an enlarged prostate, or benign prostatic hyperplasia (BPH).

Your prostate curls around your urethra, the tube that carries urine out of your body. That's why an enlarged prostate can cause frequent urination during the night, difficulty urinating, frequent daytime urination, or dribbling. By age 75, about half of all men have these symptoms, but that doesn't mean they're inevitable. If you haven't developed BPH yet, there are things you can do to avoid it.

To find out if foods could help, Italian scientists examined the diets and prostate health of more than 2,500 men. They found that the more onions or garlic the men ate, the less likely they were to get BPH. Although nobody knows exactly what causes BPH, free radicals are among the prime suspects. Experts think these cell-damaging molecules cause tissue damage that enlarges the prostate and triggers BPH symptoms. Some even think free radical damage to your cholesterol may contribute to the problem.

If that's true, perhaps the antioxidants in onions can help stop free radicals and protect your prostate from damage. More research is needed to know for sure. In the meantime, why not eat a few more helpings of onions each week — and try leeks, too. They contain many of the same healthful compounds as onions. You have nothing to lose but time in the bathroom.

Outwit high blood sugar

Studies suggest eating onions may help you control your blood sugar, which rises when you don't have enough insulin. When you eat onions, you get a compound called allyl propyl disulfide (APDS.) APDS may help prevent your body's natural deactivation of insulin, so it's tougher to run low. The extra insulin helps move blood sugar out of your bloodstream and into your cells, lowering your blood sugar level.

Clean with onions and leeks

Onions and leeks can help you clean your grill — as well as your favorite pewter and brass items. Here's how.

- You can make your own brass cleaner from an onion, but be sure you open your kitchen doors and windows to keep the room well-ventilated. Chop an onion into a small pan of water. Bring to a boil, put the lid on, and let simmer for up to two hours. Strain out the onions, dip a soft cloth in the onion water, and use it to polish brass. When you're happy with the results, wash and dry each item.

- Cleaning pewter is even easier. Just rub the pewter with the leaf of a raw leek. Rinse the item, dry it, and enjoy its new tarnish-free sheen.

- Clean your charcoal grill grate without stinky chemicals. Heat up the grill and plunge a fork into the top of an onion half. Use it as a scrub brush. Rub it up and down the grate to remove any gunk.

No-sweat way to build stronger bones

The onion is probably the last thing that comes to mind when you think of foods that can boost your bones. Yet, Swiss experts say onions may contain a secret weapon to help prevent bone loss. Strangely enough, their discovery started with a gourmet dinner for rats. To see if onions could help fight bone loss, the scientists spiced up regular rat chow with onions — and it worked. The rats rate of bone loss slowed down. Laboratory testing showed that the onion compound, gamma-L-glutamyl-trans-S-1-propenyl-L-cysteine sulfoxide (GPCS) deserves the credit. GPCS causes cells that remove old bone to get lazy and do less work. That's important because these bone robbers almost seem to work overtime in older adults.

You might not realize it but you get a completely new skeleton about once every 10 years. This happens because cells called osteoclasts constantly remove old bone, while cells called osteoblasts add new bone in its place. By the time 10 years go by, nearly every bit of old bone has been replaced. When you're young, you make more bone than you lose, and your bones get stronger. As you grow older, you make less bone, while the osteoclasts keep removing just as much bone as they always have. The result — you lose more bone than you make. If GPCS causes a work slowdown among the osteoclasts, you lose less bone.

Unfortunately, you'd have to eat nearly 14 ounces of onions a day to get the same amount of GPCS as the onion-eating rats in the study. Scientists say more research is needed to find out whether it really takes the entire 14 ounces of onions to slow bone loss. For best results, eat onions in addition to foods high in calcium and vitamin D, like dairy products. You'll be making your meals tastier and more nutritious, while strengthening your bones.

Passion fruit

Get passionate about stopping heart disease

You eat citrus fruit to get vitamin C, but after a while, an orange-a-day gets boring. Try passion fruit — a mouthwatering superfruit that oozes with vitamin C and many other heart-healthy nutrients.

Passion fruit gets its name from the plant's flower, which reminds some people of the Passion of Christ because it resembles a crown of thorns. Passion fruit, also called granadilla, is a tropical fruit long used in folk medicine. People in Brazil use it to make a heart tonic, and for good reason. Passion fruit does three terrific things for your heart and blood vessels.

Heads off heart disease. A long-term study of health professionals found that people who ate more fruits and vegetables — especially those with lots of vitamin C — have a lower risk of heart disease. Even getting just one extra serving a day made a difference. One cup of purple passion fruit has 118 percent of the vitamin C you need every day.

Strikes out against stroke. Vitamin C also helps you sidestep stroke, as one study of about 20,000 middle-age men and women revealed. The people with more vitamin C in their blood had less chance of suffering a stroke during the study. The researchers aren't sure how vitamin C helps. Some experts think a high blood level of vitamin C indicates a healthy lifestyle, which includes eating lots of fruits and vegetables.

Battles high blood pressure. Even more exciting, studies on both rats and people found that an extract made from the peel of purple passion fruit lowered high blood pressure. More than 86 percent of the people who took the extract brought down their blood pressure an average of 31 millimeters of mercury (mm Hg) systolic, the top number, and 25 mm Hg diastolic, the bottom number. Experts think something in passion fruit changes the level of nitric oxide in your blood. Nitric oxide, produced by cells inside your blood vessels, helps keep them wide open, which lowers blood pressure. A cup of passion fruit also gives you nearly a quarter of the potassium you need every day. Potassium helps reduce the effects of sodium in your body.

Trade in tomatoes for an exotic fruit

Eating more lycopene-rich foods, like tomatoes, may help prevent prostate cancer. But what if you don't like tomatoes or you can't handle eating spicy tomato sauce? Chow down on passion fruit. New research shows passion fruit is a great source of this powerful antioxidant. When passion fruit is not in season, look for apricots or watermelon to get your lycopene.

'C' how passion fruit protects your health

Switch from drinking orange juice to passion fruit juice every morning, and you'll still get a heaping helping of vitamin C. That's because a cup of purple passion fruit juice has 74 milligrams of vitamin C — nearly as much as a cup of OJ. Just look at all the ways vitamin C keeps you healthy.

Improves your odds against cataracts. Passion fruit's plentiful antioxidants, especially vitamin C, makes it a powerful weapon against cataracts. These cloudy areas of the eye's lens form when proteins clump together and block light. Damaging free radicals — from toxins, exposure to ultraviolet light, smoking, and other causes — can spur cataracts to develop. That's where antioxidants, like vitamin C, come to the rescue. They work to neutralize dangerous free radicals. According to studies in Spain and Japan, people who get lots of vitamin C from food have less risk of developing cataracts as they age. Steer clear of antioxidant supplements. Evidence suggests taking high doses may be harmful.

Boosts your immunity. Vitamin C probably won't help you get over the sniffling, sneezing, and misery of a cold once you have one. But if you take vitamin C before you get sick, you may recover more quickly. What's more, it could help keep you from getting sick in the first place. Vitamin C works especially well for people living in difficult conditions, such as very cold climates, or doing strenuous activities, like long-distance running.

Reawakens tired skin. Vitamin C is important for your body to build collagen, the connective tissue that helps wounds heal and keeps your skin looking youthful. This important vitamin also keeps a lid on free radical damage, which can weaken collagen and allow your skin to show its age. A study of middle-age women found that those who got more vitamin C in their diets had fewer wrinkles and less dry skin. That's another great reason to drink passion fruit juice.

Melt off pounds painlessly

Turn off your craving for sweets without indulging in high-calorie goodies. Try an easy pantry weight loss secret — substitution. Eat a sweet-tasting fruit, such as passion fruit or juice, instead of cookies or apple pie. You'll take in fewer calories, but you'll still stop your craving. The best advice from weight loss experts is to substitute a food that tastes similar to what you crave.

Here's how cravings work. A natural chemical made in your brain, neuropeptide Y (NPY), causes your body to crave carbohydrates. This happens at times of stress, when your body wants more fuel, and when you wake up in the morning. It's very difficult to ignore the demands of NPY, as any dieter will tell you. Instead, substitute a less energy-dense food. Fruits with natural sugars provide most of their energy in the form of carbohydrates. But one-half cup of passion fruit has 115 calories — a much better choice than a slice of homemade apple pie, which tips the scales at 411 calories.

Research shows people tend to eat about the same volume of food every day, whether it's high or low in calories. Choose low-calorie foods, like fruits and vegetables, and you're ahead of the game. In fact, a major study revealed that women who eat more fruits and vegetables reduce their risk of obesity and weight gain by 24 percent. That's good news, since people tend to gain weight as they age.

Passion fruit offers two other important benefits.

- 59 percent of the vitamin C you need in a one-half cup serving. Studies show you need vitamin C in your blood to help your body burn fat.

- 12 grams of fiber in one-half cup. Eating foods high in fiber will fill you up so you won't overeat. You'll also be less hungry between meals.

Breathe easy with tropical treatment

You may think of asthma as a children's disease, but it's not just for the young. Older adults often develop asthma. And when they do, it's more difficult to treat because they frequently have other health problems. There's also a risk of drug interactions.

People with asthma have episodes when their airways narrow, making it difficult to breathe. This is caused by both inflammation of airway linings and oversensitivity to particles in the air. An attack may include wheezing, shortness of breath, a feeling of tightness in the chest, coughing, and fast heartbeat. A serious asthma attack can kill if it's not treated promptly.

Fortunately, you can get help naturally by calling on the powerful protection of passion fruit. The passion fruit plant is used in a traditional Brazilian remedy for breathing problems, like asthma, bronchitis, and whooping cough. The connection may be passion fruit's generous amount of vitamin C. A British study determined that getting more fruit — especially with lots of vitamin C — in your diet lowers your chances of developing asthma. One cup of purple passion fruit gives you 118 percent of the vitamin C you need in a day.

Recent research shows passion fruit does a particularly good job of protecting your lungs. People with asthma who took an extract of purple passion fruit peel every day for four weeks fared better than those who took a placebo, or sugar pill. The extract improved wheezing, coughing, and shortness of breath for those who took it. The researchers suspect antioxidants in passion fruit helped calm inflammation, while flavonoids — natural plant chemicals — blocked histamine. Histamine, a chemical released by your immune system during an allergic reaction, causes inflammation.

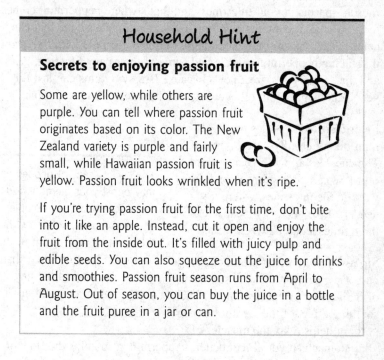

Household Hint

Secrets to enjoying passion fruit

Some are yellow, while others are purple. You can tell where passion fruit originates based on its color. The New Zealand variety is purple and fairly small, while Hawaiian passion fruit is yellow. Passion fruit looks wrinkled when it's ripe.

If you're trying passion fruit for the first time, don't bite into it like an apple. Instead, cut it open and enjoy the fruit from the inside out. It's filled with juicy pulp and edible seeds. You can also squeeze out the juice for drinks and smoothies. Passion fruit season runs from April to August. Out of season, you can buy the juice in a bottle and the fruit puree in a jar or can.

Peppermint

Soothe your insides with peppermint power

Get relief from indigestion and the painful symptoms of irritable bowel syndrome (IBS) with a chip off the old candy stick.

Calm muscle spasms. If you suffer from IBS, you may have to watch what you eat to control your symptoms. Even when you're careful, you may still have problems after a meal. Abdominal pain comes from muscle spasms in your intestines, and that's where peppermint comes to the rescue. It contains menthol, a mild natural anesthetic that can calm muscle spasms and block pain. Studies of people with IBS show that taking peppermint oil relieved some of their pain, bloating, gas, and diarrhea. That's great news because IBS symptoms can last for years, and peppermint oil is considered harmless for most people.

Enteric-coated capsules of peppermint oil are usually used to treat IBS. The capsules allow the peppermint oil to bypass your stomach and do its work in the intestines, where it's needed. Take one or two capsules three times a day between meals.

The sweet scent of peppermint may boost your memory and make you more alert. People who took memory tests with the scent of peppermint in the background scored better than those who smelled the herb ylang-ylang or no scent at all.

Sip away your upset stomach. Try a cup of peppermint tea to ease a bout of indigestion or upset stomach. The soothing effect of the menthol in peppermint helps relax the muscles of your stomach so you'll feel better. Peppermint also helps the flow of bile, which allows fats to digest. You can brew up a cup with one to two teaspoons of dried peppermint leaf, steeping it for about five minutes. Sipping peppermint tea may also relax your muscles to cure a bout of hiccups.

But don't try a peppermint cure if you have heartburn from gastro-esophageal reflux disease (GERD). Peppermint may relax muscles in your esophagus to make your heartburn even worse.

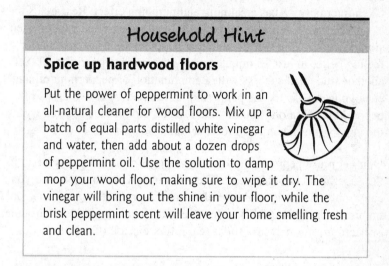

Household Hint

Spice up hardwood floors

Put the power of peppermint to work in an all-natural cleaner for wood floors. Mix up a batch of equal parts distilled white vinegar and water, then add about a dozen drops of peppermint oil. Use the solution to damp mop your wood floor, making sure to wipe it dry. The vinegar will bring out the shine in your floor, while the brisk peppermint scent will leave your home smelling fresh and clean.

Cool remedy for pain

The same herb that's the source of holiday candy canes can put an end to your aches. It works because of the plant's powerful potential to block some nerves and stimulate others. You could say peppermint cools the pain.

Power out pain. Peppermint's secret weapon is menthol, a natural anesthetic. Menthol is also used in some pain-relief creams and patches like Bengay and Icy Hot. It works by stimulating the nerves that sense cold — that's why peppermint tastes cool — and blocking the nerves that sense pain. The effect doesn't work for long, but you may get some relief.

Traditionally, people inhaled peppermint for respiratory problems and coughs. Now you can suck on peppermint candy or a cough lozenge with menthol, or sip a cup of peppermint tea to soothe your sore throat or cough. Experts believe the menthol in peppermint blocks the pain and stops the irritation that makes you cough.

Head off a headache. Peppermint oil — applied to your forehead, not taken internally — has a calming and numbing effect. Research shows it works as well as acetaminophen (Tylenol) to ease the pain of a tension headache. One study found that people with headaches started feeling better in just 15 minutes when they used peppermint oil. Yet another study had success with a combination of peppermint oil and eucalyptus oil. To try the peppermint oil remedy, put two drops of peppermint oil in one cup of water, soak a cloth in the scented water, then apply it as a compress to your forehead.

Don't confuse peppermint oil with the peppermint extract you buy in the supermarket to bake with. The oil is more concentrated, and you can usually find it in health-food or natural-product stores. You should not use peppermint oil if you have a hiatal hernia, gallbladder trouble, or heartburn from gastroesophageal reflux disease (GERD).

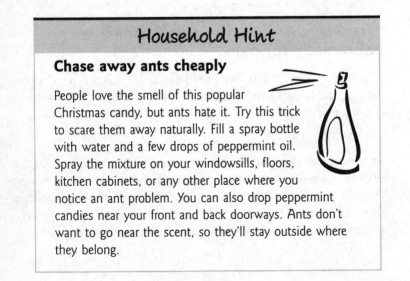

Household Hint

Chase away ants cheaply

People love the smell of this popular Christmas candy, but ants hate it. Try this trick to scare them away naturally. Fill a spray bottle with water and a few drops of peppermint oil. Spray the mixture on your windowsills, floors, kitchen cabinets, or any other place where you notice an ant problem. You can also drop peppermint candies near your front and back doorways. Ants don't want to go near the scent, so they'll stay outside where they belong.

Plums

Enjoy a plum-powerful cancer fighter

Vegetables like carrots and broccoli are full of cancer-fighting nutrients called antioxidants that help protect your cells from damage. But if you really want serious cancer protection, try a sweet, juicy plum. It's packed with five times more antioxidant power than either of those nutritious veggies. Here's the proof.

Scientists have created a system called the Oxygen Radical Absorbance Capacity (ORAC) score to measure antioxidants in foods. A higher number is better since that means a food provides more cancer-busting antioxidant strength. That's where plums really shine. A serving of 100 grams (g) of plums — about one and a half pieces of fruit — has an ORAC score of 9,240. The same amount of raw carrots has an ORAC of 1,462, while the ORAC score for broccoli is 1,844. Both veggie numbers are quite respectable as ORAC scores go, but the plum score is still five times higher than either.

Research on plums shows the ORAC comparisons ring true when your cells get a taste of the fruit. A study in Japan found that an extract of prunes, which are dried plums, worked against colon cancer cells in the lab. The prune extract caused the cancer cells to commit suicide. Experts think a certain antioxidant in the prunes, chlorogenic acid, may be responsible for this cancer-fighting effect.

Prune extract and fresh plum juice both stopped disease-causing bacteria from growing on meat in a recent study. The plum products killed 90 percent of the *E. coli* bacteria in a pound of ground beef.

To get the best cancer-busting boost, hold off eating your plums until they're very ripe. Some fruits have more antioxidants as they ripen, turning from green to other colors just like autumn leaves. That's because chlorophyll, which makes fruits green, eventually turns into antioxidant compounds called nonfluorescent chlorophyll catabolites (NCCs). NCCs mean riper is better for you.

Need regularity? Skip the prune juice

Your grandmother drank prune juice to treat constipation. You can do better. Grab a bag of dried plums — also known as prunes — and you have a more powerful remedy in hand.

As with many other fruits, the whole dried plum is better for you in many ways than its juice. In this case, prunes give you more fiber to keep your digestion regular. In fact, one-half cup of prunes has 6 grams (g) of fiber — that's twice the fiber with nearly the same calories as a cup of prune juice. Doctors recommend adults over 50 aim for 20 to 30 g of fiber every day to stay regular.

Prunes and plums also bring sorbitol to the table. This natural plant sugar behaves like a laxative, and again prunes have double the amount that's in prune juice.

Strong bones deserve proven protection

Don't let your bones turn into brittle sponges, ready to break under a tiny bit of pressure. Prevent osteoporosis with plums and prunes, great-tasting treats that are packed with bone-saving nutrients.

Post-menopausal women are most at risk of bone breaks and other problems from osteoporosis. That's why researchers focused on older women to see how eating dried plums could help. One group of women ate 12 dried plums every day, while another group ate about the same amount of dried apples. Dried plums seemed to increase their levels of a protein related to bone formation, while eating apples didn't have this benefit. The women didn't gain weight after three months on the prune diet, even though they were eating more calories. Researchers think the extra fiber in prunes helped balance things out.

Plums pack in several minerals that boost your bones.

- **Boron.** This trace mineral helps your body absorb calcium from food. Then your bones can hold on to the calcium they already have.

- **Manganese.** One-half cup of prunes has 13 percent of the manganese you need every day. This mineral helps enzymes keep your bones strong rather than becoming porous.

- **Potassium.** Like two children on a seesaw, potassium and sodium must be in balance to keep calcium where it can help you. Drinking a cup of prune juice gives you one-fifth of the potassium you need in a day, which can balance out a high-salt diet.

A cup of plums also provides about 26 percent of the vitamin C you need in a day, which helps enzymes do their job. But stick with fresh because drying plums into prunes or prune juice removes much of this important vitamin.

Plum Yummy Peanut Butter Bars

Ingredients

1 cup brown sugar, packed

1/2 cup peanut butter

2 Tbsp margarine

1/2 cup 1% milk

1/4 cup egg substitute

1 tsp vanilla extract

1 cup rolled oats

1 1/2 cup white unbleached flour

1 tsp baking powder

1/2 tsp salt

1 cup dried plums

Instructions

1. Preheat oven to 350°F, and grease a 9x13-inch baking pan.

2. In mixer bowl, beat together sugar, peanut butter, and margarine on medium speed until creamy. Add milk, egg substitute, and vanilla; beat well.

3. Combine oats, flour, baking powder, and salt; add to peanut butter mixture; mix until blended. Stir in dried plums.

4. Press evenly into prepared pan; bake 24-27 minutes or until golden brown.

(Serves 32)

Nutrition Summary by Serving

103.8 Calories (27.8 calories from fat, 26.74 percent of total); 3.1 g Fats; 2.5 g Protein; 17.4 g Carbohydrates; 0.2 mg Cholesterol; 1.0 g Fiber; 88.3 mg Sodium

Pomegranate

'Forbidden fruit' cleans out your arteries

Some people think the forbidden fruit in the Garden of Eden was actually a pomegranate — not an apple. But don't forbid this luscious scarlet beauty from your diet if you want to keep your heart young and healthy. Although only the seeds and juice are edible, inside a pomegranate you'll find natural plant chemicals like polyphenols, tannins, and anthocyanins. They function as antioxidants to keep your heart healthy. Look what they can do:

Lower LDL. This "bad" cholesterol can become oxidized by free radicals, eventually forming artery-clogging plaque. The antioxidant power of pomegranate stops this damage.

Block excess defense cells. Macrophage cells, a type of defensive cells, gobble up harmful invaders in your body. As they do their job, they also bring on changes leading to hardening of the arteries. Lab studies show pomegranate juice stops these changes.

Feed your heart. Your heart muscle needs oxygen-rich blood — just like other cells in your body. When arteries get clogged, cells starve and die. One study found that antioxidants in pomegranate juice improved blood flow to heart cells in people with heart disease who were in danger of a heart attack.

Tamp down blood pressure. Doctors say you should keep your blood pressure down to prevent heart attack and stroke. Antioxidants in pomegranates help you do that. These tropical gems also give you a nice helping of potassium, which balances the effects of sodium from a high-salt diet.

Keep arteries flexible. Studies show drinking pomegranate juice may help prevent buildup of plaque and hardening of the arteries, which can lead to a stroke or heart attack. One group of people drank 8 ounces of juice every day. After a year, their arteries were healthier, resulting in improved blood flow to the heart. It just might work for you, too.

A word of caution — if you're taking prescription drugs, like statins for high cholesterol, ask your doctor if you should drink pomegranate juice. There's some evidence pomegranates, like grapefruit, may change how enzymes in your body deal with certain drugs.

A little goes a long way

Don't overdo the pomegranate juice if you're watching your weight. One cup of pomegranate juice has 160 calories. That's a lot more than other all-natural juices. A cup of unsweetened cranberry juice has 116 calories, while orange juice has just 112 calories. Drink pomegranate juice in moderation, or add a splash to cold water for a refreshing drink.

3 ways pomegranates promote good health

It's an odd little fruit to crack, but don't be afraid to cut it open and enjoy the edible seeds. This luscious fruit can protect your vision, save your memory, and release you from arthritis pain. The secret is in the antioxidants.

A fresh, whole pomegranate contains 16 percent of the vitamin C, a powerful antioxidant, you need in a day. Then again, when the juice is pasteurized, the vitamin C is destroyed. Fortunately, pomegranates have a wealth of other antioxidant phytochemicals, including polyphenols, tannins, and anthocyanins. Pomegranate juice contains up to 1 percent polyphenols — more than blueberry or cranberry juice.

These natural plant chemicals give the fruit extra power to prevent damage from free radicals, which can wreak havoc on your cells and speed up aging. In fact, pomegranates are near the top of the charts on the scale used to compare antioxidants among foods. It's called Oxygen Radical Absorbance Capacity (ORAC). One cup of pomegranate juice has an ORAC score of 5,923. That gives it triple the antioxidant power of green tea or red wine. Here's what those antioxidants do for your health.

Protect your sight. Free radical damage to the lens of your eye can bring on cataracts, or cloudiness that can block vision. Antioxidants work to neutralize those harmful free radicals. That's why researchers are looking at how antioxidants in your diet may slow or prevent cataract formation. So far, they've found that eating more fruits and vegetables, especially with lots of antioxidants, may lower your risk of developing cataracts.

Keep arthritis at bay. Antioxidants in pomegranate may also protect your joints from arthritis. They work like COX-2 inhibitor drugs — such as celecoxib (Celebrex) — to reduce inflammation. That protects cartilage cells, which safeguard the inside of joints.

Sharpen your memory. Experts think antioxidants — polyphenols in particular — may slow the progression of Alzheimer's disease. Pomegranate extract worked in lab animals to reduce the buildup of plaques in the brain. These abnormal structures are indicators of this memory-stealing condition. The mice who drank pomegranate juice had 50 percent fewer plaques, and they scored better on memory tests.

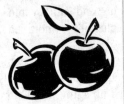
Short circuit cavities and wrinkles

Pomegranate is a traditional symbol of fertility and hope, and it may
keep you looking young. Here's why manufacturers are adding pomegranate extract to toothpaste and skin-care products.

Cleans teeth and gums naturally. Research shows pomegranate
extract, pomegranate juice, and tea — to a lesser extent — inactivates
Streptococcus mutans, the mouth bacteria that cause cavities.
Pomegranate starts working in as little as 10 minutes. Pomegranate
extract may also prevent gum disease, which hurts your chances of
keeping your teeth into old age. Researchers found that chips medicated
with both pomegranate extract and the herb gotu kola stopped gingivitis
from coming back in people treated for the condition. Look for brands
of natural toothpaste, like Life Extension, that take advantage of the
power of pomegranate.

Fights sun damage. Ultraviolet (UV) rays from the sun can lead to
wrinkles and skin cancer. But antioxidants prevent or possibly reverse

some of the damage. In fact, pomegranate — along with soy and green tea — are among the few plant products tested to see how their antioxidants battle sun damage. Pomegranate extract is even being tested in sunblock and pill form to protect your skin from damaging UV rays. For now, you can buy lotions, creams, and sunblocks that contain pomegranate extract from all-natural brands, like Burt's Bees and Murad.

Powerful pomegranate perks up potency

Pomegranate may be especially helpful for men as they age. The anthocyanidins in pomegranate juice give it great antioxidant potency. That means it may help battle both impotence and prostate cancer.

Surprisingly, trouble getting or keeping an erection may be an early sign of heart disease. That's because narrowed blood vessels can cause both heart disease and erectile dysfunction (ED), or impotence. When a man has both problems, the ED typically shows up a few years before symptoms, like chest pain, so it serves as a warning sign.

The good news is pomegranate juice may help both problems. Researchers found that men with ED who drank 8 ounces of pomegranate juice daily had less problems with impotence. They think it's because antioxidants in the juice improve blood circulation to small blood vessels.

Other research hints pomegranate may work to slow prostate cancer. Certain natural plant chemicals in pomegranate called ellagitannins are changed to ellagic acid in your body. Lab tests show they can block the growth of prostate cancer cells. Ellagitannins are the most abundant type of polyphenol in pomegranate, and they're released when you squeeze the whole fruit for juice. Secure your masculine health, and kill two birds with one glass of pomegranate juice every day.

Pomegranate Vinaigrette

Ingredients

8 oz pomegranate seeds

1/2 cup apple cider vinegar

1/2 cup honey

1 pinch salt

1 pinch pepper

1 cup olive oil

Instructions

1. Place pomegranate seeds, apple cider vinegar, honey, and seasonings in a blender. Blend thoroughly.
2. Slowly add olive oil while continuing to blend. Adjust seasonings and strain.

(Serves 8)

Nutrition Summary by Serving

325.5 Calories (243.8 calories from fat, 74.89 percent of total); 27.1 g Fats; 0.3 g Protein; 22.5 g Carbohydrates; 0.0 mg Cholesterol; 0.2 g Fiber; 3.0 mg Sodium

Potatoes

Super spuds save your heart

Maybe meat and potatoes aren't so bad, after all. Evidence is piling up that the antioxidants and complex carbohydrates in potatoes can actually lower your cholesterol, triglycerides, and overall heart disease risk.

For three weeks, researchers fed rats either a potato diet, with the natural nutrients in potatoes; a pure starch diet; or a simple sugar diet. The animals on the potato plan lowered their cholesterol and triglycerides more than 30 percent, plus boosted their levels of antioxidants, compared to the starch and sugar diets. Potatoes have three things going for them that sugar and starch lack.

- **Fiber.** Spuds specialize in a type of fiber called oligo-fructo-saccharide, or OFS for short. This fiber ferments in your large intestine, a process that produces short-chain fatty acids. These compounds, in turn, seem to squash the production of cholesterol in your liver. Add to that, fiber keeps you from absorbing some fat and sugar, which may lower your triglycerides.

- **Antioxidants.** Potatoes are rich in vitamin C, a powerful antioxidant. In fact, one baked potato provides almost a third of your daily vitamin C needs. It's also loaded with vitamin E, phenols, and the carotenoid lutein, all important antioxidants. Having enough vitamin E in your body is one key to preventing heart disease. Vitamin E helps keep your cholesterol from oxidizing, a type of damage linked to heart disease. Rats fed potatoes in this study were less likely to have their cholesterol oxidize than those fed pure starch or sugars.

- **Potassium.** You can lower high blood pressure, a major risk factor for heart disease, by eating more potassium-packed foods like potatoes. Study after study show people who get more potassium in their diets tend to have lower blood pressure, and that upping your intake helps treat high blood pressure. Just one baked potato puts you well on your way, with a quarter of the potassium you need in a day.

Many of these heart-healthy nutrients hide in the potato peel. When possible, eat the skin on boiled potatoes, or make "dirty" mashed potatoes that include the peel. You'll maximize the benefits and enjoy the extra flavor and texture.

Color offers clues to healing

You can tell what kinds of healing phytochemicals a potato contains by the color of its flesh.

- Spuds with red, blue, and purple flesh are rich in anthocyanins, known for battling heart disease and cancer.

- Orange flesh points to high levels of zeaxanthin, which guards your vision.

- Yellow-fleshed potatoes pack lots of lutein for preserving eyesight and preventing cancer.

Protect yourself from type 2 diabetes

Potatoes are a classic no-no for people with diabetes. The problem — most potatoes have a high Glycemic Index (GI), a measure of how much a food raises your blood sugar. Potatoes contain lots of easily digested starch, which can cause a quick rise in blood sugar. But it is possible to eat them and still keep a lid on your blood sugar.

For 20 years, researchers from Harvard University and Brigham and Women's Hospital studied the eating habits of a group of nearly 85,000 women. Those who ate potatoes were more likely to develop type 2 diabetes, especially if they were obese or not active. Experts think the main reason is because of their high GI. Other studies suggest eating a diet of mostly high-GI foods raises the type-2 risk between 37 and 59 percent in men and women.

Despite the scary statistics, potatoes are chock-full of many nutrients, including antioxidants, so banning them from your diet isn't a great idea, either. Luckily, you can make them healthier by lowering their GI.

- Serve cold potatoes. Boil potatoes and refrigerate overnight, then serve cold the next day. Chilled potatoes form resistant starch, which is harder to digest. This, in turn, lowers their GI and prevents a sharp rise in blood sugar after eating them.

- Dress them with vinegar. Adding a dash of vinaigrette to potatoes blunts the rise in blood sugar and insulin.

- Top off potatoes with low-fat cheddar cheese, chili, or baked beans. All of these toppings lower the GI of potatoes and other starches. Cheese has the biggest impact. In one study, adding a cup of shredded cheese dropped the GI of potatoes so much that they registered as a low-GI food.

You can boost their nutrition even further by using skim milk in mashed potatoes and fat-free sour cream to top off baked potatoes.

Cut cancer-causing compounds

Potatoes and other starchy foods can form cancerous compounds called acrylamides when cooked, but you can dodge the danger with these clever tips.

- Soak raw potatoes before cooking. That includes French fries. In a British study, soaking raw potatoes for 30 minutes cut acrylamides by 38 percent, while soaking for two hours reduced them 48 percent. Simply washing raw potatoes, on the other hand, only lowered acrylamides 23 percent.

- Add a dash of vinegar or lemon juice to the water you use to soak raw potatoes. This raises the water's pH, which helps prevent acrylamides from forming.

Experts are hard at work trying to breed high-carotenoid potatoes. Scientists have discovered the carotenoids in potatoes are the same kind found in the human eye. That means eating spuds super-rich in these plant compounds could one day help treat blinding diseases such as macular degeneration and cataracts.

- Microwave raw potato products, like French fries, before frying. Researchers found that nuking fries from 10 to 30 seconds slashed the amount of acrylamide formed during frying up to 60 percent.

- Choose course-cut over fine-cut fries. Acrylamides usually form on the surface of potatoes. Less surface area means fewer acrylamides.

- Fry potatoes and fries at temperatures no higher than 175 degrees. Also, fry or bake your potatoes only until they turn golden yellow. Overcooking and high temperatures create more acrylamides.

- Don't store spuds in the refrigerator. The cold causes sugars to form in potatoes. The more sugar a potato packs, the more acrylamides you get when you cook it. Store them in a dark, dry, cool but not cold location — about 50 degrees — with good ventilation.

Cold potatoes defeat gut diseases

Potatoes are an easy food to digest for people suffering from irritable bowel syndrome, and now research shows they may actually protect your gut from diseases.

Raw potatoes and cold, boiled potatoes contain resistant starch. This type of fiber won't break down in your small intestine, so it travels to your large intestine where it ferments, producing butyric acid and other compounds. Researchers fed pigs a diet heavy on raw potatoes for 14 weeks and discovered important gut changes compared to pigs eating corn starch.

Eating resistant starch seems to:

- protect the lining of your gut against attacks by bacteria and other harmful organisms.

- create bulky stool, which protects against compounds that can irritate your gut or cause cancer.

- squash the overreaction of the immune system in your gut, which may ease inflammatory bowel diseases (IBD), including colitis.

- boost levels of butyrate, a compound formed from the fermentation of resistant starch. Butyrate may help prevent the growth of abnormal, pre-cancerous cells in the colon.

You can get more resistant starch by eating boiled potatoes cold instead of hot, and from foods such as legumes, green bananas, pasta, and cereal.

Powdered milk

Cooking trick builds better bones

Your doctor says you aren't getting enough calcium to protect your bones even though you eat several servings of calcium-rich foods every day. Never fear. Here's a nifty trick that not only adds calcium to your diet, but helps your body absorb more of it. Add a little powdered milk to your recipes.

A tablespoon of nonfat powdered milk has around 60 mg calcium. So you'll get more calcium in your diet just by adding powdered milk to dishes you eat every day. Experiment with cream sauces, stews, casseroles, muffin recipes, soup mixes, cookie recipes and, of course, mashed potatoes. A quarter cup also adds around 100 calories, 15 grams of sugar, and 160 mg salt to a dish, so take that into consideration when planning your meals.

If you choose a nonfat powdered milk fortified with vitamin D, your body will absorb more of the calcium in both the powdered milk and the foods you add it to. That's because your body needs vitamin D to help absorb calcium. And if you're one of the 30 to 60 percent of people who don't get enough vitamin D, you need that extra boost to benefit from all the calcium you take in. While powdered milk won't guarantee a full day's helping of calcium and vitamin D, it will help you close in on the recommended amounts. And that might make the difference between bones that fracture easily and bones that stay strong for years to come.

Household Hint

Enjoy home-grown veggies for less

Spend less money on your garden and harvest more delicious vegetables. Here's how.

- Add powdered milk to the water you use to give your tomatoes a drink, and they'll reward you with the juiciest-tasting crop you've had yet. What's more, the calcium in this common pantry product thwarts blossom end rot so you don't have to throw out as many tomatoes.

- Use powdered milk to store extra seeds. Corn and onion seeds can last one year while seeds for tomatoes, beans, lettuce, and carrots last up to three years. But they'll sprout unless they're kept quite dry. Powdered milk makes a good drying agent, so simply store your seeds in a closed jar with some freshly bought powdered milk. Just be sure to store the jar in a dark, cool place, and change the powdered milk every six months.

Shore up your body's defenses

Adding powdered milk to your recipes gives you more than extra vitamin D and calcium. It helps protect against serious problems that can have long-term effects on your health.

Reinforce your smile. Periodontitis is a gum disease that makes people lose their teeth, and you're more likely to get it if you're running low on calcium, studies say. Consider these examples.

- Research from Sri Lanka found that people aged 70 and older have a higher risk of worsening periodontitis if they have low blood levels of calcium.

- People under age 70 also had higher odds of periodontal disease if they had a low calcium intake, reported a study from the State University of New York. In fact, women who got less than 500 mg of calcium from their diets were 54 percent more likely to get periodontitis than women who got at least 800 mg of calcium a day.

How can calcium make such a difference? Periodontitis gets its start when bacteria build up between your teeth and gums. Over time, these bacteria can invade and wear down the bone and tissues that support your teeth until your teeth have nothing left to cling to. But if you get enough calcium, the jaw bone becomes tougher and more difficult for bacteria to break down. And that may be enough to hold off periodontitis and keep your teeth firmly attached.

"D"-feat an early danger. The -itis in periodontitis means inflammation is part of the problem. It shows up as one of the most common problems dentists encounter — chronic gingivitis. This inflammation of your gums is caused by the same bacteria and plaque that give you cavities. But, in some people, gingivitis gradually destroys the ligament and bone supporting the teeth, and periodontitis sets in. Powdered milk delivers a nutrient that can help — vitamin D. Boston University researchers discovered that people with the highest blood levels of vitamin D were less likely to show signs of gingivitis than people who had the lowest blood levels. The researchers think this vitamin helps fight inflammation. And just as controlling a small fire prevents a big blaze, controlling the early inflammation of gingivitis may prevent periodontitis.

Turn back heart attack risk. The deaths of journalist Tim Russert and actor Don S. Davis are a sad reminder of how sudden and dangerous heart attacks can be. But believe it or not, fending off gum disease may help you avoid a similar fate. Nine out of 10 people with heart disease also have severe gum disease, one study reports. Some experts think this happens because the bacteria that cause plaque and gum disease sneak into your bloodstream and make plaque in your arteries. Others think the inflammation in your gums can lead to inflammation in your arteries. Either problem could lead to a heart attack or stroke, so your best bet is to prevent them both. Taking advantage of the calcium and vitamin D in powdered milk is one easy way to shore up your body's defenses.

Household Hint

Save money with two natural cleansers

Cut costs with these easy replacements for makeup remover and silver polish.

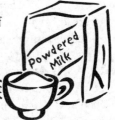

- Remove makeup with a spoonful of powdered milk mixed with some warm water. Just dab it on with a cotton ball, and rinse.

- Forget smelly silver cleaners with all their chemicals. Instead, mix a tablespoon of lemon juice and 5 ounces of powdered milk into 1 1/2 cups of water. Soak your silver in this potion for six hours and then rinse. Dry thoroughly and enjoy the fresh shine.

Tropical Low-Fat Fruit Smoothie

Ingredients

1 cup papayas, chopped

1 cup mangoes, chopped

1 cup fresh pineapple, chopped

1/2 cup water

1/2 cup ice cubes

2 Tbsp sugar

1 tsp vanilla extract

1 1/3 cup dry nonfat milk

Instructions

Place all ingredients in a blender, cover, and blend until smooth.

(Serves 4)

Nutrition Summary by Serving

231.4 Calories (4.6 calories from fat, 2.01 percent of total); 0.5 g Fats; 15.1 g Protein; 42.6 g Carbohydrates; 8.0 mg Cholesterol; 1.9 g Fiber; 228.8 mg Sodium

Probiotics

Boost immunity with beneficial 'bugs'

Probiotics from yogurt and other foods may help you stay well during cold and flu season. Oddly enough, the secret to this success may lie in your gut instead of your nose. One of the best-kept secrets of your immune system is gut-associated lymphoid tissue (GALT). GALT is found in organs throughout your digestive tract and makes up nearly 70 percent of your immune system. But the real excitement begins when GALT meets helpful bacteria called probiotics.

Probiotics are dynamic disease fighters with anti-inflammatory powers, and they deliver more health benefits than basic nutrition alone. When these "good bugs" find GALT, they make your immune system rev up its defense tactics and churn out immune-boosting compounds. Not only does this help you fight off stomach flu and other digestive ills, but studies like these suggest probiotics can do much more.

- Factory employees who drank a probiotic supplement daily for nearly 12 weeks had one-third fewer sick days, a Swedish study reports. The probiotic in the supplement was *L. reuteri*, the same friendly bacteria you'll find in Stonyfield Farm yogurt at your grocery store.

- Spanish researchers discovered that volunteers who avoided probiotic foods for several weeks showed signs of reduced immunity, but just eating probiotic products or yogurt with live and active cultures revitalized their immune responses.

- A mere three weeks of drinking milk fermented with yogurt cultures and *L. casei* reduced the length of respiratory infections, like colds, in older adults, Italian researchers say. The yogurt also shortened the course of infections of the digestive tract. You can get *L. casei* by drinking DanActive.

For the most health benefits, try probiotic products like DanActive dairy drink or Stonyfield Farm yogurt. These contain some of the same probiotics used in the studies, so they may help you stay healthier during cold and flu season. If you have suppressed immunity, talk to your doctor before trying probiotics.

Household Hint

Choose the best probiotic every time

Probiotics are fast becoming the
rock stars of the food world.
Instead of just finding them
in yogurt and milk, now you
can get them from specialty
cheese, cereal, supplements, and
even juice — plus more probiotic foods are coming soon. To be sure you get real probiotic benefits, you
must choose your products wisely. Here's how to start.

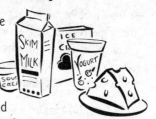

- Look for the expiration date. If the number of organisms is listed on the product label, that's the number
  living when the product was made. Unfortunately, far
  fewer of those probiotics may be living when you buy
  it. Exposure to heat, moisture, and oxygen can reduce
  the probiotics in a product, so buy as far ahead of the
  expiration date as you can.

- Check yogurt labels for the National Yogurt
  Association seal or the words "live and active cultures" to make sure you get viable probiotics.

- Experts say you need 1 billion to 10 billion good bacteria
  a day. If you read the labels on supplements, these
  amounts may be written as "1 x 109" or "109" for 1 billion units, and "1 x 1010" or "1010" for 10 billion units."
  ConsumerLab tests supplements to make sure they contain all the probiotics promised on their labels, and they
  are free of dangerous contaminants. Visit their Web site
  at *www.consumerlab.com* to find out which brands
  deliver the goods — and which ones don't.

Chew your way out of cavities

A new probiotic chewing gum may help you avoid cavities and expensive dental work. Developed by a German company called BASF, this chewing gum contains the newly discovered probiotic called *L. anti-caries*. It helps fight the cavity-causing bacteria, *Streptococcus mutans (S. Mutans)*.

These trouble-making bacteria stick to the surface of your teeth and spew out harsh acid that causes tooth decay. But *L. anti-caries* makes all the little *S. Mutans* clump together like raisins in a box. That means they can't cling to your teeth because they're too busy clinging to each other. Tests show chewing probiotic gum cuts the number of bacteria in your mouth to a tiny fraction of what was there before — and that helps keep you cavity free. This new gum is coming to stores soon.

New diabetes fighter protects your heart

Guests in India may be offered dahi, a yogurt-type dish, with griddle-fried bread or mixed with rice. This probiotic-rich food may be just what they need to help control blood sugar and guard against heart attack.

Diabetes tends to get worse over time, but recently, researchers from India's National Dairy Institute discovered evidence that dahi and its probiotics may slow diabetes' progress. In a study of animals at high risk for diabetes, they found that animals who ate no dahi experienced a higher rise in blood sugar over the long haul than dahi eaters.

Dahi eaters also took significantly longer to develop glucose intolerance, a sign that diabetes is setting in. In fact, the researchers say probiotics are probably the reason dahi delayed glucose intolerance several times longer than milk. But that's not the only protection these probiotics offer. Three out of four people with diabetes die from heart disease or its complications. In the study, dahi probiotics helped put the brakes on heart attack risk factors, like total cholesterol and "bad" LDL cholesterol.

Future research may reveal whether dahi has the same effects on people as on animals. Meanwhile, why not add probiotics to your diet. The dahi in the study contained *L. casei* and *L. acidophilus*. You don't have to travel to India to find them. You can get them from Stonyfield Farm yogurt, and you may find them in other products, too. Just remember, some probiotic products contain added sugars, so talk to your doctor about which one is right for you.

Pick probiotics that keep their promises

Look for these names on the labels of foods, drinks, and supplements. According to ConsumerLab, these probiotics have the most research behind them. More research means they're more likely to deliver what they promise.

- *L. acidophilus*
- *L. casei*
- *L. gasseri*
- *L. bulgaricus*
- *B. bifidum*
- *B. lactis*
- *B. longum*
- *Saccharomyces boulardii*

Other promising probiotics include *L. reuteri*, *B. infantis*, *L. johnsonii*, *L. rhamnosus*, *B. breve*, and *Streptococcus salivarius*.

Relieve IBS symptoms at last

Probiotics could make irritable bowel syndrome (IBS) a thing of the past. These helpful "bugs" show promise in combating IBS symptoms, like diarrhea, constipation, pain, and gas. Plus, they're easier to tolerate than IBS medicines. In fact, these friendly bacteria have shown so much potential that companies are studying new probiotics to specifically target IBS. Consider these studies on Activia yogurt and the new Align supplement.

- A large study of adults with constipation as the main symptom of IBS found that *B. animalis DN-173 010* twice daily improved discomfort, bloating, and regularity. This version of *B. animalis* is the probiotic in Activia yogurt.

- People with any type of IBS who took *B. infantis* saw a modest improvement in all IBS symptoms. *B. infantis* is the probiotic in Align.

Probiotic products like these may help because they work like ladybugs. Just as any good garden has ladybugs and plant-eating pests, your digestive system has several hundred species of probiotics and harmful bacteria. Normally, probiotics help keep harmful bacteria in check, just like ladybugs control pests in your garden. However, a round of antibiotics, a bout of food poisoning, or various illnesses can kill a lot of your good bacteria. That leaves the harmful bacteria free to be fruitful and multiply. When too many harmful bacteria take over your digestive system, they can cause the gas, bloating, diarrhea, and constipation of IBS.

Adding probiotics from yogurt or other probiotic products may restore your bacterial balance and improve your IBS symptoms. It may also suppress low-grade inflammation in your bowel lining that may make IBS pain worse. Keep in mind, probiotics aren't like antibiotics. A single round of probiotics won't cure your IBS the way antibiotics cure an infection. You only get the symptom-stopping effects of these friendly bacteria for as long as you keep taking them.

If you'd like to try probiotics for your IBS symptoms, talk to your doctor first. If she approves, try Activia or another yogurt containing live, active cultures. Not only are they cheaper than prescription medicines, they're also easier to swallow and much more delicious. If you can't tolerate yogurt, ask your pharmacist how to get the Align supplement.

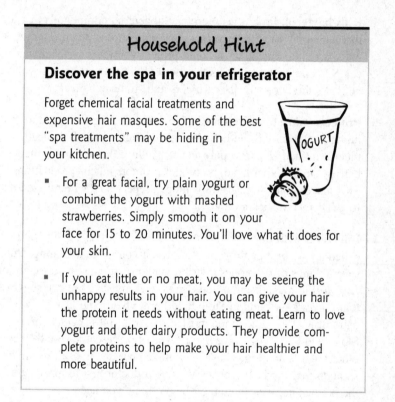

Household Hint

Discover the spa in your refrigerator

Forget chemical facial treatments and expensive hair masques. Some of the best "spa treatments" may be hiding in your kitchen.

- For a great facial, try plain yogurt or combine the yogurt with mashed strawberries. Simply smooth it on your face for 15 to 20 minutes. You'll love what it does for your skin.

- If you eat little or no meat, you may be seeing the unhappy results in your hair. You can give your hair the protein it needs without eating meat. Learn to love yogurt and other dairy products. They provide complete proteins to help make your hair healthier and more beautiful.

Beat stubborn ulcers for good

Probiotics can help you avoid ulcers, painful gastritis, and perhaps even stomach cancer. That's because bacteria called *Helicobacter pylori (H. pylori)* help cause these problems, and studies suggest probiotics help reduce your *H. pylori* population. In fact, scientists think probiotics may fight the dangers of *H. pylori* in at least four ways.

■ **Tames inflammation.** If you feel like you've got a fire in your belly, *H. pylori* may be the reason why. Your immune system responds to *H. pylori* by unleashing a small army of inflammation-causing compounds that can cause pain. Probiotics thin down this army, so you get less inflammation and less misery.

■ **Kills bacteria.** Probiotics secrete antibacterial compounds that act like bug spray to help keep *H. pylori* populations down. That may not sound like much, but it could protect you from stomach cancer. Some research suggests the more *H. pylori* you have in your body, the higher your risk of ulcers and stomach cancer.

■ **Protects your stomach lining.** *H. pylori* can cling to your stomach lining more easily if the lining isn't producing as much protective mucus. In fact, *H. pylori* may actually reduce the stomach's mucus barrier. On the other hand, probiotics promote mucus production. This makes your stomach walls more slippery so it's literally harder for *H. pylori* to stick around.

■ **Interferes with bacterial colonies.** *H. pylori* needs a compound called urease or it can't form colonies on your stomach lining. But several kinds of probiotics interfere with urease, making it tough for *H. pylori* to make itself at home in your stomach. Research suggests that *L. casei* — found in Stonyfield Farm yogurt and DanActive dairy drink — is among the most successful. But *L. reuteri* from Stonyfield Farm yogurt may work well, too. Research results using other yogurts and foods have been mixed but that doesn't mean you shouldn't try them. Just check with your doctor first to make sure the product delivers enough of the probiotic you need.

Unfortunately, studies show probiotics can't eliminate *H. pylori* or ulcers all by themselves. To get rid of them, you'll need your doctor's help. Even then, probiotics can make things easier. The antibiotic doctors often prescribe to wipe out *H. pylori* may have side effects, like diarrhea, nausea, and vomiting. Research suggests adding probiotics can help ease these side effects.

And in those rare cases where a first round of antibiotics fails to eliminate *H. pylori*, probiotics can still help. Taiwan researchers found that people who tried four weeks of a special probiotic yogurt were more likely to wipe out *H. pylori* with their second round of antibiotics. If your doctor ever prescribes antibiotics for an ulcer, be sure to ask about taking probiotics, too.

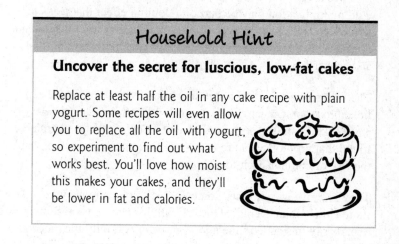

Household Hint

Uncover the secret for luscious, low-fat cakes

Replace at least half the oil in any cake recipe with plain yogurt. Some recipes will even allow you to replace all the oil with yogurt, so experiment to find out what works best. You'll love how moist this makes your cakes, and they'll be lower in fat and calories.

5 ways to sidestep colon cancer

Colon cancer makes an appearance a little like putting a car together on an assembly line. A chain of events must happen in the right order to produce a car. Likewise, colon cancer depends on a chain of events, too. If one of those things doesn't happen, you may avoid colon cancer completely. That may be where probiotics come in. These "good bugs" can throw a monkey wrench into the process of forming colon tumors. Here's how.

■ They hamper cancer-causing enzymes. Some of your body's natural enzymes, like beta-glucuronidase and nitroreductase, can help cancer-causing compounds to form. Fortunately, some probiotics hamper these enzymes and that may be enough to prevent the harmful compounds from developing. Studies suggest two of these probiotics are *L. casei* Shirota — available from Yakult probiotic drink — and *L. acidophilus* found in acidophilus milk and yogurts.

- They prevent changes to normal cells. Faulty changes to more than 20 of the genes in your normal cells can cause colon cancer. Studies show probiotics help your body resist compounds that try to make cancer-causing changes to your genes.

- They lower bile acid. Too much bile acid along the colon wall can make cells reproduce too fast, like adding gasoline to a fire. This wild multiplication may be part of a domino effect that leads to tumors. Research suggests probiotics may help restrict the amount of bile acid in your bowel, so your cell production stays normal and cancer free.

- They reduce inflammation. Inflammation in the bowel has been linked to colon cancer risk in people with inflammatory bowel diseases, like Crohn's disease and ulcerative colitis. Yet, research has found that probiotics can reduce the inflammation — and perhaps the risk of colon cancer, too.

- They improve transit time. Some people's colons move waste more slowly than average. Doctors call this slow transit. Some experts say this added time allows more opportunity for cancer-causing toxins to form. But studies show probiotics can help reduce the time waste spends in slow-transit colons, which may prevent tumor-causing toxins, too.

No human studies have proven that probiotics can prevent cancer, but animal and laboratory studies seem to suggest probiotics can help. Besides, research suggests 70 percent of colon cancer cases aren't hereditary. That means the choices you make every day can help you avoid this dangerous cancer. So give probiotics a try. You might be very glad you did.

Ward off IBD flare-ups

A new probiotic might help you resist surprise flare-ups of diarrhea and other symptoms of inflammatory bowel disease (IBD). This yeast, called *Saccharomyces boulardii (S. boulardii)*, may be just what you need to keep Crohn's disease or ulcerative colitis under control.

When medical treatments start controlling the symptoms of IBD, doctors say it is "in remission." Unfortunately, remission isn't guaranteed to last and may end suddenly when you least expect it. But a combination of 1 gram of *S. boulardii* with the drug mesalamine every day kept more people in remission from Crohn's disease than mesalamine alone, a small study found.

Another study hinted that 750 milligrams (mg) of *S. boulardii* a day might prevent a relapse in people with ulcerative colitis who are in remission. Scientists suspect this probiotic may squelch production of an inflammation-promoting chemical in the gut. Since inflammation is what causes the symptoms of colitis, dowsing it may help fight IBD symptoms as well.

Other probiotics, such as VSL#3 and Mutaflor, have also shown promise against IBD. Talk to your doctor before you try *S. boulardii* to be sure it's the best probiotic for you. If your doctor approves of *S. boulardii*, you won't need a prescription. Just ask your pharmacist for Florastor, a behind-the-counter probiotic that contains *S. boulardii*. Other brands might also be available, so shop around to get the best price.

Protein

Powerful protection from chicken soup

Sometimes old wives' tales aren't just tales. For example, chicken soup has been scientifically proven to help you fight off the miserable symptoms of a common cold. It has not one but three weapons to help put you on the road to recovery.

- When a cold virus attacks, virus-killing "hit men" called neutrophils gang up and fight back. But instead of just killing the virus, they also trigger inflammation in your airways. This can cause a chain reaction that stirs up cold symptoms and makes you miserable. Stephen Rennard, a lung disease specialist at the University of Nebraska Medical Center, tested various chicken soups and discovered the secret to their powerful defense. The soup causes fewer neutrophils to gang up, which translates to less inflammation and milder cold symptoms.

- The protein in chicken contains compounds that act a little like medicines. For example, cysteine is an amino acid unleashed while chicken is cooking. This amino acid is similar to acetylcysteine — a mucous-thinning drug used against bronchitis.

- Research shows that sipping this soup hot can help clear up congestion, keep you hydrated, and ease the pain of a sore throat. Both the steam and the liquid from the soup can help you heal.

Fight back against weak muscles

Nearly one out of two Americans over age 60 has sarcopenia — a condition that may put you at risk for disability, obesity, and type 2 diabetes. It could even take away your independence. But many people have discovered they can put the brakes on sarcopenia — and you can, too.

Simply put, sarcopenia is the natural loss of muscle strength and muscle mass as you age. It may seem harmless, but here are four reasons why you should take it seriously.

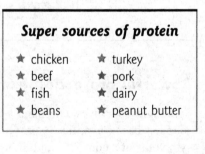

Super sources of protein

★ chicken ★ turkey
★ beef ★ pork
★ fish ★ dairy
★ beans ★ peanut butter

- Sarcopenia that barely affects you in your forties can make walking, climbing stairs, and keeping up with your family difficult as you grow older.

- Muscle helps you burn calories, so losing muscle means you burn fewer calories and gain weight more easily.

- Having less muscle may also be linked to insulin resistance — an early sign of diabetes.

- Resistance from your muscles helps maintain the strength of your bones. That's why doctors often recommend weight-bearing exercises to help fend off osteoporosis. They know that less muscle means less power to protect your bones.

Eat the right amount of protein. Neither sarcopenia nor its scary consequences are inevitable. In fact, a recent small study found that elderly adults who ate a 4-ounce beef meal built as much muscle over the next few hours as "kids" in their 30s and 40s. However, as few as 30 percent of older adults eat the minimum recommended amount of protein every day, so they may not be getting the fuel needed to help slow muscle loss.

Fortunately, this problem can be fixed. To figure out how much protein your body needs, whip out your calculator, and multiply your weight in pounds times .36. If you weigh 200 pounds, you should aim for 72 grams of protein daily. At 125, you'll only need 45 grams of protein a day. This may sound like a lot, but you can get 25 grams of protein just by eating a serving of chicken breast or turkey no larger than a deck of cards. A similar-sized serving of salmon or canned tuna delivers more than 20 grams of protein, and many other fish are protein-rich as well. Other good sources of protein include peanut butter, dairy foods, nuts, lean beef, and pork.

Pump up your protection. Strong muscles need help from the outside as well as the inside. Ask your doctor about strength training programs for people in your age group. Research suggests that simple resistance exercises can help you hang on to more muscle power as you age. Keeping your muscles strong will help you control your weight as well as fend off other diseases, like osteoporosis and diabetes. It could also mean more years of walking, stair climbing, keeping up with your family, and keeping your independence.

Household Hint

Shrink your grocery bill

The average American spends nearly one-fourth of his annual grocery bill on four proteins — meat, poultry, fish, and eggs. The prices of these items recently rose nearly 5 percent in just one year, and they're expected to go even higher. Slash spending on groceries with these tips.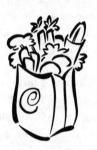

- Make a list. USDA research touts this as the #1 money saver for anyone on a limited budget. For even better results, plan your menus for the week first. Impulse buys may account for 40 to 60 percent of your grocery bill, experts say.

- Buy what you need. Ask the staff in your meat department if they can package a smaller cut of meat to match the amount you need. Or have them tenderize a cheaper "tough cut" of meat for you.

- Adjust your menu. If meat costs are straining your food budget, eating smaller portions of meat — and larger amounts of cheap protein like beans — will help shrink your grocery bill even more.

Melt off pounds the easy way

You'll keep your hunger pangs at bay and shed pounds more easily if you include protein in your diet. Science offers three good reasons why you need protein when you're trying to lose weight.

- It's better at suppressing the appetite-causing hormone ghrelin than fats or carbohydrates, according to a University of Washington study. That may help squelch your hunger and cut your calorie intake.

- It helps your body burn more calories.

- It increases the amount of fat you lose and helps you retain lean muscle.

Moderation is best. That doesn't mean you should go overboard. A small New York study found that people who ate moderate amounts of protein lost about as much weight and body fat in three months as people who ate a high-protein diet. What's more, a Purdue University expert says that just one 3-ounce serving of lean protein can be enough to make a difference in your appetite during the day. A 3-ounce serving of lean beef, turkey, or chicken breast is about the size of a deck of cards, so that's not much food. For best results, use this protein to replace a high-calorie, low-protein food that's currently in your diet.

Timing is important. You'll get more bang for your protein buck if you eat your protein early in the day. A St. Louis University study compared women who ate a high-protein egg breakfast with women who ate a bagel and cream cheese. Although both breakfasts contained the same amount of calories, egg eaters took in fewer total calories over the next day and a half. Egg eaters also took longer to become hungry again.

Don't forget about carbs. Focusing on protein doesn't mean you should avoid carbohydrates. A small University of Washington study found that women who ate a high-protein, average-carb, low-fat diet for 14 weeks said they weren't as hungry as when they ate less protein. Yet they still lost weight. They also cut their daily food intake by 450 calories — even when they were told to eat as much as they wanted. But you won't find a fried chicken dinner in this diet. The trick, say the researchers, is to choose lean or low-fat forms of protein.

Get the right amount. Talk to your doctor before adding extra protein to your diet. Because you will cut calories, your protein requirements will differ from what you normally need. While trying to lose weight, aim for the recommended daily allowance of 46 grams per day for women or 56 grams for men. But some people may need a different goal. For example, adding too much meat to your diet may also add enough trans fats and saturated fats to increase your risk for heart disease, stroke, and cancer. In addition, adding too much protein may be dangerous for people who have kidney problems. So if you're at high risk for conditions like these, get you doctor's advice on the best protein goal for you.

Get hormone-free meat without the high organic price by buying chicken instead of beef. Chickens aren't given growth hormones because it's against the law.

Surprising secret to healthy joints

You may be at higher risk for osteoarthritis if other people in your family already have it. Along with exercising and watching your weight, include some protein in your diet. It may give your joints added protection.

Experts say you need reasonable amounts of protein in your diet to keep your joints healthy. Why? Proteins are made up of amino acids, and your body can use these amino acids to form healthier joints. You may especially benefit from sulfur-based amino acids like the cysteine you get from chicken soup. Animal studies suggest a possible link between osteoarthritis and low levels of sulfur in the joints. Fortunately, eating protein-rich foods may supply the amino acids you need so your joints can flourish.

If you have already developed osteoarthritis, you may need to be picky about which proteins you eat. Some experts think dairy products, shrimp, peanuts, red meats, and poultry may aggravate the condition. Talk to your doctor to learn more.

Practice cancer-free grilling

You gave up fried meats because they were bad for your heart, and now experts say grilled and broiled meats may raise your risk of cancer and other diseases. But that doesn't mean you can't ever eat meat or use your grill. You just have to know how to do it properly.

- Speed up your grilling. Pre-cook the meat in the microwave for one minute. This removes most of the compounds that form cancer-causing heterocyclic amines (HCAs.)

- Become a frequent flipper. High-heat cooking helps create HCAs and disease-causing advanced glycation end products (AGEs). Flipping meat keeps the cooking temperature lower.

- Marinate your food. Marinades protect against the grill's high temperatures so fewer HCAs can form.

Red grapes

Fruit of the vine protects your heart

How do French people get away with eating rich diets of butter-filled pastries and heavy sauces, yet keep their hearts young and healthy? The answer to this "French paradox" may be in the glass of red wine that accompanies their dinners.

Grapes — along with juice and wine made from them — contain natural plant chemicals that help your heart, including antioxidant polyphenols like resveratrol, quercetin, anthocyanins, and catechin. Both grape skins and flesh have powerful antioxidants, but resveratrol — important for your heart in many ways — is mostly in grape skin. That's why so much resveratrol ends up in purple grape juice and red wine.

These phytochemicals are nothing to sneeze at. In fact, your refrigerator could be holding more healing power than the big drug companies' labs. Here's how nutrients in grapes can benefit your heart.

Bring down high blood pressure. When your blood pressure is up, it's like you've put your fingers over the end of a garden hose. Your blood is moving with more force, making your heart work harder. That can lead to a heart attack, stroke, heart failure, or other problems.

But studies show grape juice can lower your blood pressure. Research in Korea found that men with high blood pressure who drank Concord grape juice every day for eight weeks improved their conditions. Both blood pressure numbers — systolic and diastolic — were lower. Experts credit grape juice flavonoids. These antioxidants cause cells to produce more nitric oxide, which relaxes blood vessel walls. That means lower blood pressure and less danger of other heart problems.

Cancel out excess cholesterol. Nutrients in grapes also may improve your cholesterol levels, another marker for possible heart problems. One study found flavonoids in grape juice lowered LDL, sometimes called "bad" cholesterol, while raising HDL, or "good" cholesterol. These improvements remained for weeks after people in the test stopped drinking grape juice.

Battle inflammation. These same phytochemicals also cut back on inflammation, a sign you may be at risk for clogged arteries and a heart attack. But women who got more flavonoids from the foods they ate — including apples, pears, and red wine — had a lower risk of heart disease.

You can get your grape nutrients from red wine, but don't overdo it. Experts say one glass a day may help, but two or more glasses simply add stress to your circulatory system. You can also buy supplements of resveratrol, but they're not well regulated. Besides, there's more to grape goodness than a single nutrient — you need the whole bunch.

Sweet path to a better memory

Nearly half of women in their 90s have dementia. That's a scary future, but you can do something to hold on to your memories. Boost your brainpower as you age with the natural compounds in grape juice.

Grapes are like tiny packages of blockbuster nutrition. They contain several phytochemicals — natural plant chemicals — that work as antioxidants to preserve your memory. Antioxidants like proanthocyanidins, epicatechin, and resveratrol fight oxidation, a cell damaging process that may play a role in Alzheimer's disease (AD), a common form of dementia.

Squeeze grapes for juice or wine, and the best nutrients come along for the ride. In fact, people who drink more juices like grape juice are well on their way to avoiding AD as they age. In one study, volunteers who drank three or more glasses of juice a week could reduce the risk of this memory-stealing disease by 76 percent. All types of fruit and vegetable juice were counted in that study, but some may work better than others. Researchers at the University of Glasgow measured the antioxidants in 13 fruit juices and found that purple grape juice had the highest concentration. So grape juice may be your best bet for a younger brain.

The truth behind dark raisins

Raisins won't help if you're trying to add more heart-healthy resveratrol to your plate. Most raisins — even the dark ones — are made from white grapes, typically the Thompson Seedless variety. That means they had little resveratrol to begin with. Even more is lost during processing. But don't cross raisins off your snack list just yet. They are a great source of other nutrients like fiber, potassium, and boron. Plus they taste great.

Go purple to battle cancer

Darker is better when it comes to preventing cancer. That's because the phytochemicals that give grapes their power also give them their brilliant color. These powerhouses, called anthocyanins, do the same for blueberries and blackberries.

Studies show anthocyanins in grape juice may help fight breast cancer by protecting DNA from cancer-causing compounds. Changes in DNA — the tiny material that carries your genetic code — allow cells to grow out of control into tumors. Researchers tested anthocyanins to prevent colon cancer as well, since these phytochemicals are easily absorbed in your digestive tract. Anthocyanins slowed the growth of colon cancer cells while leaving healthy cells alone.

What works in the lab must also be tested in the real world. In this case, it worked. One study found that people who drink more than three glasses of red wine every week have a lower risk of colon cancer. Scientists give some of the credit to the other heavy-hitting phytochemical in grapes, resveratrol. This antioxidant also changes how breast cancer cells react to estrogens, which can bring on tumor growth. Add a little resveratrol, and this harmful process slows down or even stops.

Resveratrol works in a similar way to battle prostate cancer in men. This time, however, it's male hormones that are affected. But resveratrol managed to slow or stop tumor growth without changing testosterone levels in mice who were tested with the phytochemical. These results brought great excitement to Dr. Coral Lamartiniere, the University of Alabama at Birmingham scientist who oversaw the study.

"A cancer prevention researcher lives for these days when they can make that kind of finding," he said.

Listen up for 'grape' news

Resveratrol, a phytochemical found in abundance in grape skins, may protect your hearing as you age. The major cause of age-related hearing loss is damage from a lifetime of loud noises. But research has found that rats fed resveratrol suffered less hearing damage when they were exposed to loud noises. Oxygen free radicals can destroy the delicate hairs of the inner ear, responsible for picking up sound waves. The antioxidant powers of resveratrol prevent this damage and preserve your hearing.

Fight diabetes with a fabulous fruit

Food is on your mind a lot when you're battling diabetes — or even if you're simply watching your weight. Either way, you can benefit from eating grapes a-plenty. They have resveratrol, a natural plant chemical that does three great things to help control diabetes and battle the bulge.

Keeps a lid on blood sugar. People with diabetes have to watch what they eat and perhaps use insulin to keep their blood sugar balanced. Resveratrol can help in part by stimulating your cells to take sugar out of the blood while lessening the effects of oxidation, thus helping to maintain balance.

Soothes diabetic pain. Trouble keeping your blood sugar stable can lead to nerve damage. You'll know it because of the pain and numbness in your legs and feet. It's called diabetic neuropathy, and there's not too much doctors can do for this pain, short of suggesting medications. But resveratrol comes to the rescue, cutting the pain by blocking the pain receptors that transmit it. Mice with diabetes got sweet relief from diabetic pain with a daily dose of resveratrol.

Stifles new fat cells. Whether or not you have diabetes, excess weight may be an issue. Several studies show resveratrol can help in this battle of the bulge. Researchers in Germany found that pre-fat cells — targeted to turn into fat-storage cells in your body — don't develop when resveratrol is in the mix. Resveratrol may also function in the same way a low-calorie diet works to keep your body from aging too fast. Yet you don't have to give up eating what you love.

Red wine has lots of resveratrol, but it may not be right for you if you have diabetes. The American Diabetes Association cautions people with diabetes to drink alcohol in moderation and be careful of how it may affect your blood sugar. Grape juice may be a better choice.

Household Hint

Natural way to dye cloth

Try this easy method of dyeing fabric next time you need to keep your grandchildren busy for an afternoon. You'll end up with lovely purple cloth for crafts or home-decorating projects. You'll need:

2 large cans frozen grape juice

4 Tbsp salt

4 cans water

1/4-yard pieces of unbleached cotton fabric

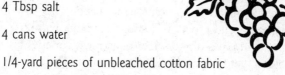

If you want to use fresh grapes, pick a variety like Concord grapes, which have dark skins and flesh. Use about a pound of grapes for a pound of fabric. Mix together the ingredients and bring to a boil. Simmer until you see a deep color, about one hour. Let the water cool, then strain it if you're using fresh grapes.

Pour this dye concentrate into a large enameled pan, and add enough water to cover your fabric. Add wet cloth. Simmer the fabric and dye for at least one hour, stirring occasionally, until the fabric is a shade darker than you want. Rinse the fabric in cold water until it runs clear, then hang it to dry.

Stomp out disease-causing bacteria

Know why berries have resveratrol? To keep the plants safe from fungus. That same natural plant chemical works with other grape compounds to help fight off the bacteria that cause cavities, food poisoning, and even stomach ulcers.

Experts have long known that red and white wines — even with the alcohol removed — can kill *S. mutans* bacteria, the bugs that lead to tooth decay. Wine also kills the bacteria that cause many sore throats, *S. pyogenes.* One theory was that acids in the wine keep the harmful bacteria from growing.

New research shows resveratrol and catechins — another kind of plant chemical in grapes — work against *H. pylori,* bacteria that can live in your stomach and make you more prone to ulcers. They also kill *E. coli,* a major culprit in food poisoning, and other harmful germs. A study using several types of red wine found most varieties killed these harmful bacteria, yet left probiotic bacteria alone. These are helpful bacteria your body needs for good digestion and other functions. Enjoy grapes in all their forms to get these bacteria-busting effects.

Resistant starch

Little-known nutrient nixes colon cancer

A special starch in everyday foods can turn the tables on colon cancer. You probably eat it already and don't even realize it. Resistant starch, in foods like green bananas, cold pasta, and coarsely milled grains, doesn't digest like other starches. Instead of breaking down in your small intestine, it passes through to your colon, where it ferments. This makes it more similar to fiber.

That's great news for your colon. Resistant starch sweeps away cells with damaged DNA — cells that might otherwise turn cancerous.

And, like fiber, it adds bulk to stool and moves it more quickly through your digestive tract, so cancer-causing substances have less contact with your gut.

Plus, it nurtures the growth of friendly bacteria in your colon. These bacteria lower the pH level inside your colon and produce short-chain fatty acids, such as butyrate, which squash cancer growth. Butyrate, the main food for healthy colon cells, prevents the growth of cancer in lab studies. It may even help kill damaged colon cells before they turn cancerous.

Meat lovers should eat plenty of resistant starch. The protein in meat also ferments in your colon, but it produces potentially toxic compounds, including ammonia. In fact, research shows the amount of protein you eat can influence the development of colon cancer. Pumping up your protein increases the DNA damage to colon cells in animal studies, which contributes to cancer growth. Eating foods rich in resistant starch, like cold, boiled potatoes and cold pastas, shrinks this link by reducing DNA damage.

Special snacks battle high blood sugar

Snack bars made with resistant starch (RS) make a safe, tasty, between-meal bite for people with diabetes. These treats make perfect daytime snacks when you need something that won't send your blood sugar through the roof. Thanks to their resistant starch, you get a healthy dose of carbs that give you a gradual, sustained rise in blood sugar, rather than a sharp spike. RS bars are best eaten in place of regular snacks that have fast-digesting carbohydrates. Look for "maltodextrin" in the ingredient list — a code word for resistant starch.

Easy way to burn fat and halt hunger

Not all carbohydrates are alike. Some are actually good for melting away fat, controlling appetite, and improving insulin sensitivity. The problem is, people eat the wrong types of carbs. Most store-bought foods contain carbs that are easy to digest. But carbs that digest slowly, such as resistant starch (RS), can help you in several ways.

Burn more fat. Getting just 5 percent of your daily carbs as resistant starch helps you burn an incredible 20 percent more fat, especially around your buttocks. This special starch ferments in your colon, producing compounds called short-chain fatty acids (SCFAs). These cause your liver to burn body fat for fuel. Best of all, the effect is long-lasting, and you don't have to make major changes to your diet.

Satisfy your hunger. New evidence shows resistant starch may help regulate your appetite by affecting the hormone leptin, which switches off your hunger signal. Researchers put 20 rats on a diet low in RS, and 20 on a diet rich in RS. The low-RS mice stopped responding to leptin, while the rats on the high-RS diet seemed more satisfied after meals.

Super sources of resistant starch

- ★ green bananas
- ★ cold, boiled potatoes
- ★ puffed wheat cereal
- ★ pumpernickel bread
- ★ cold pasta
- ★ white beans
- ★ lentils
- ★ muesli

Store less fat. What's more, the low-RS rats packed on more body fat, even though the rats on the high-RS diet ate more food. The low-RS rats also had larger fat cells, a trait linked to poor insulin sensitivity. Resistant starch seems to change how the body stores fat. The SCFAs it produces help control the growth and spread of fat cells.

That means adding more resistant starch to your diet could keep you from putting on fat, plus help control your blood sugar and insulin levels naturally. You can get more RS simply by making smart food choices. Replace the starchy foods you normally eat with those high in resistant starch. For instance, serve pasta and potatoes cold instead of hot — chilling them produces resistant starch. Buy bananas green instead of ripe. Green bananas contain resistant starch.

Rosemary

Tasty way to preserve your memories

"There's rosemary, that's for remembrance," says Hamlet's sweetheart during her mad speech near the end of Shakespeare's famous play. Crazy as she was, Ophelia was right. The fragrant herb rosemary may help you keep your memories.

Rosemary is a favorite cooking and healing herb, long used to help digestion and enhance memory. You'll find it growing as a silvery evergreen shrub, and bees just love it. Its strong antioxidant powers may help preserve memory by stopping the breakdown of acetylcholine, an important brain chemical. Acetylcholine carries messages along nerves, so it's important for your brain to function correctly.

Researchers in California and Japan worked together to figure out exactly how rosemary protects your brain. They identified carnosic acid, an antioxidant in rosemary that prevents free radical damage to cells. Experts think this kind of damage contributes to Alzheimer's disease and normal age-related forgetfulness. The great thing about carnosic acid is it stays inactive, waiting until it's needed. The presence of dangerous free radicals causes carnosic acid to become active to defend your cells against damage. This same antioxidant may also protect your brain from stroke injury.

Herbs that heal

Find out what herbal remedy works best for common health problems. Be careful to avoid herbs you may be allergic to, and talk to your doctor about how a specific herb may interact with drugs you take.

Herb	Condition or symptoms	How it works
aloe vera	constipation	juice made from the plant's dried latex has a laxative effect
cayenne	high cholesterol, weight loss, back pain (topical)	capsaicin in peppers has antioxidant effect to lower cholesterol, makes you feel full faster so you eat less, topical use stops body chemical "substance P" from transmitting pain
chamomile	insomnia	up to three cups of chamomile tea daily has a mild sedative effect
cinnamon	diabetes	works like insulin to change proteins that affect blood sugar and lower inflammation
curcumin	diabetes	curcumin in turmeric, the spice that makes curry yellow, helps control blood sugar
feverfew	migraine headaches	dilates small blood vessels to improve blood flow and prevent or relieve headache
flaxseed	constipation	contains both soluble and insoluble fiber — 3 grams total per serving — to keep bowels moving
garlic	blood clots	allicin and pyruvate in garlic break down fibrin in blood to prevent clotting
ginger	arthritis, motion sickness	may work like an anti-inflammatory by inhibiting COX-2, acts on brain chemical receptors to block motion sickness
ginkgo biloba	memory	contains antioxidant flavonoids to battle cell damage, improve blood flow in brain

Herb	Condition or symptoms	How it works
ginseng	diabetes	ginsenoside in ginseng lowers blood sugar and works as an antioxidant to block eye and kidney damage
lavender	mood, anxiety	lavender aromatherapy improves mood and relieves anxiety
marjoram	stress, high blood pressure, insomnia	dilates blood vessels when used in massage oil, scent calms and relaxes in a marjoram-lavender bath
oregano	food poisoning	phytochemicals in oregano stop the growth of *L. monocytogenes*, a food bacteria; works even better when mixed with cranberry extract
parsley	rheumatoid arthritis (RA)	high vitamin C content prevents inflammatory polyarthritis, or RA in multiple joints
peppermint	irritable bowel syndrome (IBS)	peppermint oil in enteric-coated capsule slows activity of intestinal smooth muscles to relieve IBS, worsens heartburn by relaxing muscles in esophagus
psyllium	constipation, high cholesterol	soluble fiber forms gel in intestines to move waste and soften stool, slows absorption of fats from food
rosemary	cancer, memory loss	blocks cancer-causing compounds from forming during cooking of meat and carbohydrates, carnosic acid in rosemary works as an antioxidant to protect brain cells
sage	mood, memory	essential oil and dried sage leaf boost memory and mood, may have antioxidant effect on brain enzymes
St. John's wort	depression	when taken regularly, it may relieve depression better than some antidepressant drugs
willow bark	osteoarthritis, back pain	contains salicylates for anti-inflammatory and pain-relieving effects similar to aspirin

Aromatic way to condition your hair

You can find everything you need for gorgeous hair and a healthier scalp in the fresh herb section of your grocery store. Start with a handful of rosemary and sage leaves and crush them to release their oils. Put the leaves in a pot with two cups of water. Bring to a boil, and simmer for a few minutes. Remove the pot from the heat, and let the leaves steep for three hours. Strain out the leaves, pour the liquid into a spray bottle, and store it in the refrigerator for up to a week. Spritz the mixture on dry hair until it's thoroughly wet. Massage it into your scalp and don't rinse. Your hair will be shiny and soft, smelling as fresh as an herb garden.

If you're battling alopecia areata — patchy hair loss that is different from typical male pattern baldness — researchers have good news for you. One study found a mixture of rosemary oil and other essential oils — including thyme, lavender, and cedarwood — slowed hair loss. People with alopecia areata had good results when they massaged the oil mixture into their scalps daily for seven months. The essential oils worked much better than the carrier oil used as a placebo.

Household Hint

Learn to love multi-talented rosemary

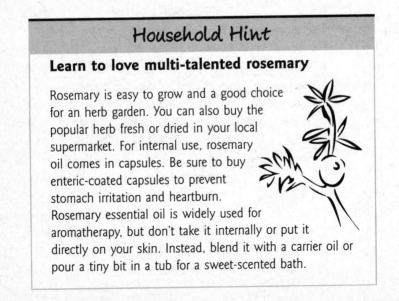

Rosemary is easy to grow and a good choice for an herb garden. You can also buy the popular herb fresh or dried in your local supermarket. For internal use, rosemary oil comes in capsules. Be sure to buy enteric-coated capsules to prevent stomach irritation and heartburn. Rosemary essential oil is widely used for aromatherapy, but don't take it internally or put it directly on your skin. Instead, blend it with a carrier oil or pour a tiny bit in a tub for a sweet-scented bath.

Roasted Potatoes with Rosemary

Ingredients

1 lb. Russet potatoes, approximately 3 cups cubed

2 tsp canola oil

1/2 tsp rosemary, dried

1/2 tsp salt

Instructions

1. Preheat the oven to 450°F.

2. Coat a baking sheet with vegetable cooking spray.

3. Wash and peel the potatoes.

4. Cut the potatoes into 1-inch cubes, and put them in a large bowl.

5. Put the oil, rosemary, and salt in a small bowl. Stir together.

6. Pour the oil mixture over the potatoes. Stir to coat the potatoes evenly.

7. Spread the potatoes on the baking sheet.

8. Bake for 25 to 30 minutes, or until lightly browned.

Serves 6

Nutrition Summary by Serving

73.5 Calories (14.3 calories from fat, 19.46 percent of total); 1.6 g Fats; 1.6 g Protein; 13.7 g Carbohydrates; 0.0 mg Cholesterol; 1.0 g Fiber; 200.3 mg Sodium

3 unusual ways to stay healthy

Rosemary may be your body's best friend when it comes to cutting down on cancer-causing compounds in cooked food. You may have heard of the dangers caused by acrylamides in cooked foods.

Acrylamides are created when carbohydrate-rich foods are cooked at high temperatures — baked, fried, or grilled. Experts think they may cause cancer, and french fries, bread, and chips are major sources. But research shows rosemary may stop this reaction. Adding rosemary to bread dough before baking lowered the amount of acrylamides in bread by close to 60 percent. While some research shows acrylamides may not increase cancer risk, it can't hurt to play it safe.

Rosemary also may help keep cooked meat safe. When meat is grilled at a high temperature, cancer-causing compounds called heterocyclic amines (HCAs) can form. Adding rosemary to the meat before cooking was shown to lower the amount of dangerous HCAs formed, this time by up to 72 percent. Researchers think antioxidants in the rosemary are responsible.

As if that's not enough, rosemary offers another way to keep your food safe. It kills certain bacteria that can cause food poisoning, including *E. coli*. Because the herb adds a fragrant touch and woody flavor when you roast it with meat or mix it into bread dough, cooking with rosemary is a delicious way to better health.

Salba

Chia: secret weapon in heart disease

Dust off your chia pet. Those tiny seeds are turning out to be powerful weapons in the fight against heart disease and type 2 diabetes.

Edible chia seed, a close relative of those furry, fast-growing plants, was once a favorite grain of ancient Aztecs. Now it's poised for a comeback. Growers have bred a special variety of chia seed called salba, which shows huge promise against diabetes and heart disease.

Salba boasts more fiber and heart-healthy alpha-linolenic acid (ALA), a type of polyunsaturated fatty acid (PUFA), than any other natural food. Plus, it's an excellent source of calcium, protein, magnesium, and iron and packs more antioxidants than some berries — all nutrients linked to a lower risk of heart disease.

People with diabetes may benefit most from the resurgence of chia seeds and salba. Three out of four people with diabetes die from heart-related problems. No surprise, since seven out of 10 have high blood pressure, a major risk factor for heart disease. Thanks to new research, experts think sprinkling salba on food can improve those odds.

Cap high blood pressure. In a Canadian study, 20 people with type 2 diabetes added either salba or another whole grain to their regular meals. After 12 weeks, salba-eaters enjoyed 20 percent lower blood pressure.

Experts think your body converts the vast amounts of ALA in salba into another PUFA, eicosapentaenoic acid (EPA). It uses EPA to make compounds called prostaglandins. Most prostaglandins trigger inflammation in your body, but the ones made from EPA help counter it. They don't cause your blood vessels to narrow as much as other prostaglandins. Wider, more relaxed blood vessels mean lower blood pressure.

Quell inflammation. Another compound, called C-reactive protein (CRP), helps doctors measure your inflammation levels. More CRP means more inflammation in blood vessels, and a greater likelihood of heart disease.

While salba didn't lower people's levels of high-sensitivity CRP, the other grain in the experiment raised their levels dramatically. By the study's end, salba-eaters had levels 40 percent lower than the non-salba group. What's more, the more ALA and EPA people had in their bloodstream, the lower their CRP dropped.

Prevent blood clots. Salba also dropped levels of two substances that help blood clot — von Willebrand factor and fibrinogen. Too much of either can boost your risk of heart disease, especially if you have diabetes.

Beat the big three. In rat studies, nibbling on whole chia seeds lowered their triglycerides while ground seeds raised their good HDL cholesterol. What's more, chia seeds fed to rats on high-sugar diets kept them from developing insulin resistance and problems with cholesterol and triglycerides, plus improved these conditions in rats who already had them. Chia even seemed to trim belly fat in rats on the high-sugar diet.

Besides being loaded with heart-guarding nutrients, salba can also help you meet your whole grain goals each day. That's important, because eating just three servings of whole grains daily may slash your risk of heart disease and diabetes. Unfortunately, the main sources of whole grains in your diet — bread and breakfast cereals — are usually so heavily processed that they are stripped of their nutrients.

Egg-cellent way to cut bad fat

Eggs enriched with heart-healthy omega-3 fats are about to get even better for you. Poultry farmers feed ground flaxseed to hens to get eggs with an extra dose of omega-3. But chia seeds may produce even healthier eggs, since they pack more omega-3 than flaxseed or any other grain.

Feeding chia seed to hens produced eggs with less cholesterol and saturated fat and more polyunsaturated fat, particularly omega-3. Cooked chicken benefits, too. Feeding chia to broiler chicks trimmed the saturated fat but boosted the good, alpha-linolenic fatty acid (ALA) in both white and dark meat — all without changing the taste.

Salba is different. It's a whole grain you can sprinkle directly on yogurt, salad, soup, and other foods, and a little goes a long way. Less than 1.5 ounces of dried, edible chia seed equals two full servings of whole grains. You can enjoy the seeds whole or ground. Keep salba and chia seeds in your refrigerator to protect their fragile, friendly fats.

Chicken Salad with Salba

Ingredients

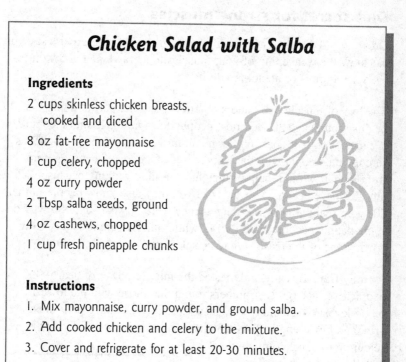

2 cups skinless chicken breasts, cooked and diced

8 oz fat-free mayonnaise

1 cup celery, chopped

4 oz curry powder

2 Tbsp salba seeds, ground

4 oz cashews, chopped

1 cup fresh pineapple chunks

Instructions

1. Mix mayonnaise, curry powder, and ground salba.

2. Add cooked chicken and celery to the mixture.

3. Cover and refrigerate for at least 20-30 minutes.

4. Add pineapple chunks and chopped cashew nuts before serving.

(Serves 6)

Nutrition Summary by Serving

313.0 Calories (140.9 calories from fat, 45.02 percent of total); 15.7 g Fats; 20.9 g Protein; 27.8 g Carbohydrates; 43.4 mg Cholesterol; 10.1 g Fiber; 463.5 mg Sodium

Selenium

Diet secret for strong muscles

Growing old does not necessarily mean growing frail. Experts say you can slow the weakening of your muscles to a crawl, and you won't even need drugs or doctors to do it.

The loss of muscle mass and strength is a natural part of aging that begins around age 30, but most people don't notice it until a couple of decades later. If it goes too far, it can turn into a condition known as sarcopenia. People with the worst cases of sarcopenia can't get up from a chair without help or may have trouble walking because their muscles have become so weak. Yet you may also know people in their 80s who seem almost as strong as they were 20 years ago. So why do some people become terribly frail while others seem to barely slow down? One of the reasons may be selenium.

A study from Tuscany, Italy tested the muscle power of nearly 900 people over age 65. Researchers found that those with the lowest blood levels of selenium were also more likely to have poor knee, grip, and hip strength. This may happen because your body needs selenium to make compounds called selenoproteins. The Italian researchers think seleno-proteins may help protect against loss of muscle strength. While no one has proven that extra selenium guarantees more muscle, getting enough selenium

Super sources of selenium	
★ barley	★ Brazil nuts
★ fish	★ rice
★ turkey	★ whole grains

in your diet is important. Enjoy foods like fish, rice, and a Brazil nut or two every day.

For even better results, also ask your doctor about these powerful sarcopenia stoppers.

- Protein. Many older adults don't get enough of the protein their muscles need. Fortunately fish, rice, and nuts can give you protein in addition to selenium.

- Strength training. Some experts say lifting weights — when done properly — may be the best defense against sarcopenia. These exercises won't turn you into an Olympic weight lifter, but they may give you the strength you need to continue your daily activities and keep your independence for years to come.

Simple way to sidestep cancer

Former White House press secretary Tony Snow was only 53 when he died of colon cancer. That's why it's never too early to take steps to prevent this dangerous cancer. Fortunately, something as simple as getting enough selenium in your diet can help.

Study after study has shown that death rates from cancer are higher in places where soils and people's diets are low in selenium. New research suggests that giving your body enough selenium may help you avoid colon cancer.

- University of North Carolina researchers took blood samples from people who were having colonoscopies. They learned that people with the highest blood levels of selenium were less likely to have adenomatous polyps in their colons than people with the lowest levels. Adenomatous polyps are the kind most likely to turn into cancer.

■ University of Arizona scientists went a step further. They studied people who had already had adenomatous polyps removed to see if selenium might help prevent these polyps from returning. They found that people with the highest blood levels of selenium were one-third less likely to redevelop polyps than people with low selenium levels.

So if you're worried about your risk of colon cancer, enjoy selenium-rich foods like turkey, barley, and tuna salad. And for even better results, watch your weight and exercise every day.

High selenium linked to diabetes

Too much selenium may put you at risk for diabetes. That's what a new study from Johns Hopkins University found after examining tests from more than 8,000 people. In fact, people with the highest blood levels of selenium were 57 percent more likely to have diabetes than those with the lowest levels. Another study found that people who had already developed skin cancer were 25 percent more likely to get it again if they took 200 mcg in selenium supplements every day.

But this doesn't mean you should avoid selenium. Instead, aim to get the recommended daily allowance of 55 mcg from foods. If you take a multivitamin, experts recommend choosing one that contains no more than 70 mcg of selenium a day.

Keep your joints jumping

You may have an easy way to defend your knees against painful osteoarthritis thanks to some clever scientists in North Carolina and a little-known disease in China.

The soils in some parts of China contain little or no selenium. This leads to selenium deficiencies in both the crops grown in these areas and in the people who live there. University of North Carolina researchers noticed that these same areas are famed for occurrences of Kashin-Beck disease, a rare condition that causes people to develop joint problems early in life. This gave the researchers an idea. Perhaps selenium could affect the health of your joints and cartilage enough to lower your risk of osteoarthritis.

To find out, the researchers examined the toenail clippings and knee X-rays of 940 people. Since toenails grow slowly, the clippings provided a fairly accurate record of each person's selenium levels during the previous months. Meanwhile knee X-rays helped determine which people were developing osteoarthritis, who already had it, and who were arthritis-free. The researchers found that people with the highest selenium levels were 40 percent less likely to have osteoarthritis and 50 percent less likely to have severe osteoarthritis affecting both knees.

Selenium may make a difference because of its reinforcing powers. Osteoarthritis wears away the cartilage that cushions your bones from one another. In fact, it's the thinning of that cartilage that causes the knee pain and swelling of osteoarthritis. But selenium may help strengthen that cartilage so you keep more of it for longer. As a result, you may delay the symptoms of osteoarthritis for months or years — or perhaps even avoid them completely.

Soy

Cut through cholesterol confusion

Despite all the hype surrounding soy, leading experts now say it may do little, if anything, to improve your cholesterol levels. But don't give up on tofu, yet. Eaten the right way, it may still slash your risk of heart disease.

For years, studies touted soy's ability to slash cholesterol. Unfortunately, after reviewing all the research, the American Heart Association (AHA) says soy supplements only cut bad LDL cholesterol 3 percent, despite the high dosages used. They had no effect on good HDL cholesterol or harmful triglycerides.

While it won't do much for your cholesterol, soy may improve other predictors of heart disease. Postmenopausal women who took 54 milligrams of genistein, a soy compound, daily for two years lowered their risk of heart disease, compared to women not taking genistein.

- Phytoestrogens in soy, such as genistein, make for strong antioxidants, which prevent changes in your arteries and cholesterol that can lead to atherosclerosis.

- Genistein raised women's levels of OPG, a compound that keeps calcium from building up in your blood vessels and protects the cells lining your blood vessels from dying. High OPG levels may protect against heart disease and heart-related death.

- The supplement also lowered women's fibrinogen levels, a substance in your blood that can raise your risk of heart disease. Fibrinogen tends to rise after menopause.

Although soy is no silver bullet, the AHA says soy foods can benefit your heart, because they're rich in heart friendly fats, fiber, vitamins, and minerals and low in saturated fat. Eat soy nuts and soy burgers in place of other high-protein foods that have more saturated fat and cholesterol, like red meat and full-fat dairy. Don't waste your money on soy supplements. The AHA says it's the whole package of nutrients, not just one or two, that might give your heart an edge.

Win the war on fat

Replacing fatty protein, like red meat, with soy foods may have an added bonus — weight loss. Studies show soy protein is as good as other types of protein at helping you shed pounds and maintain a healthy weight by reducing hunger and making you feel full.

Animal studies suggest soy is actually better at helping you slim down. Genistein, a soy isoflavone, may block the growth and spread of fat cells, which affect how much fat your body stores. Human studies, however, have not proven this. Experts warn loading up on soy without cutting back on calories elsewhere won't help you lose weight. Your best bet — stick to a healthy, reduced-calorie diet to drop those extra pounds.

Little legume keeps breast cancer at bay

Soy prevents breast cancer one day. The next day, it causes it. When every study says something different, it's hard to know what to believe. New research reveals which women may benefit from soy, and which women should avoid it.

As far back as 1990, the National Cancer Institute announced soy might prevent cancer. Research focused on beating breast cancer, because countries where people eat lots of soy foods, like Asia, have low rates of this disease. Unfortunately, the news wasn't all good. Many experts worried soy could actually make some women more likely to develop breast cancer. Soy compounds called isoflavones can work like estrogen in the body. That's why scientists refer to them as phytoestrogens.

Estrogen fuels the growth of certain breast tumors. Experts worry the phytoestrogens in soy may do the same thing. So far, no clear evidence shows that "outside" estrogens, like phytoestrogens, boost breast cancer risk. The estrogen your body makes has a much greater impact.

New research suggests soy may, in fact, protect against breast cancer if you eat it regularly. Out of 35,000 Chinese women, those who ate the most soy foods were 18 percent less likely to develop breast cancer. Postmenopausal women faired even better, with a 26 percent lower risk.

You don't need to eat enormous amounts of soy. Experts estimate as little as 10 milligrams (mg) of isoflavones daily — about one regular serving of tofu — should offer protection. Two servings, or 20 mg of isoflavones, may cut your risk a little more, up to 29 percent. The earlier in life women begin eating soy, the more protection they seem to gain. While experts say soy foods are safe for most women, breast cancer survivors taking a selective estrogen-receptor modulator (SERM), like tamoxifen, should avoid them and isoflavone supplements. Genistein, the main isoflavone in soy, may interfere with these drugs.

Beef up your bones

You may be able to strengthen your bones just by snacking on soy nuts, soybeans, and other soy foods. These simple legumes seem to boost bone density and strength in women after menopause.

You lose bone quickly after menopause, anywhere from 5 to 20 percent of your bone mass in the first five years alone. That's because estrogen affects how your body builds bone. Cells called osteoclasts are constantly breaking down bone and reabsorbing it. Osteoblast cells, on the other hand, build new bone. When your estrogen levels drop after menopause, the osteoclasts work faster than osteoblasts, so you lose bone faster than you can build it.

Estrogen replacement therapy was once the recommended treatment for osteoporosis. Since the dangers of hormone therapy became known, new drugs called SERMs (selective estrogen-receptor modulators) have taken its place. Then again, a natural alternative may be hiding in the health food aisle. New studies suggest plant estrogens, or phytoestrogens, in soy act like natural SERMs, affecting both osteoblasts and osteoclasts.

- Genistein, soy's main isoflavone, helps "turn off" those destructive osteoclasts.

- Daidzein, another isoflavone, gives osteoblasts a boost to form more bone.

Most studies show these isoflavones prevent bone loss in animals, but whether they work in humans is less clear. In one study, women with weak bones took supplements containing vitamin D and calcium. One group also got 54 milligrams (mg) of genistein, while the other group took a placebo, or fake pill. The genistein group had greater bone density after two years of treatment and better signs of overall bone health. The soy compound didn't cause any precancerous changes, either, the way estrogen therapy can.

A review of 10 studies found that menopausal women who ate soy had greater bone density of the spine. Women who got more than 90 mg of isoflavones daily for six months showed the greatest improvement.

These doses may sound like a lot, but they're average amounts in Asian countries where soy is a staple food. For instance, you can get

54 mg of genistein just by eating a cup of boiled soybeans and half a cup of tofu yogurt, or 2 ounces of dry roasted soy nuts and a cup of soy milk. Those same combinations put you well over 90 mg of total isoflavones, too.

How soy products are processed affects their isoflavone content. Generally, nonfermented foods, like roasted soybeans and edamame, pack two to three times more than fermented soy, such as miso and tempeh. Low-fat and nonfat soy milk contain the least. Soy flour, on the other, is a good source, and baking with it won't destroy the compounds.

Put the squeeze on lung cancer

Eating soy could drop your risk of lung cancer a whopping 44 percent. While estrogen may help lung cancer grow, phytoestrogens seem to squash it — and soy is rich in phytoestrogens. Scientists suspect these compounds crush lung cancer the same way they battle breast and prostate cancers by:

- triggering cancer cells to die.

- preventing the growth of blood vessels in tumors.

- blocking the spread of cancer to other parts of the body.

Research in both humans and mice suggest phytoestrogens work. Men who got the most soy isoflavones were 44 percent less likely to develop lung cancer. Women benefited slightly less, with a 22-percent drop in risk.

A study in mice may help explain how these compounds work. In mice with lung tumors, a soy extract slowed the growth of tumor cells and caused them to die faster than tumors in nontreated mice. Genistein, the main isoflavone in soy, seemed to neutralize proteins called Akt. Akt help tumors survive, develop a system of blood vessels to feed spreading cancer cells, and resist cancer treatments. And you don't need to stock up on expensive soy supplements. These results occurred with amounts of soy typically eaten in Japan.

Hidden isoflavones in food

Check this handy chart to see how many isoflavones you eat everyday, whether you're avoiding them or trying to boost your intake. Some of the sources may surprise you.

Food	Serving Size	Total Isoflavones (milligrams)
White beans, raw	1/2 cup	0.74
Split peas, raw	1/2 cup	2
Soybeans, mature, boiled	1/2 cup	47
Soy nuts (dry roasted soybeans)	1/2 cup	152
Soybean oil (salad or cooking)	1/2 cup	0
Soy sauce, made with soy and wheat	1 tablespoon	0.26
Soy milk	1 cup	30
Miso	1/3 cup	43
Tempeh	1/2 cup	36
Tofu	3 ounces	20
Soy cheese, cheddar	3.5 ounces	7
Soy flour, defatted	1 cup	131
Beef patty with VPP (Vegetable Protein Product), cooked	1 patty	1
Meatless (soy) hot dog	1 hot dog	11
Green Giant, Harvest Burger, Original flavor, All Vegetable Protein Patties, frozen, prepared	1 patty	8

Get a grip on menopause symptoms

Estrogen replacement therapy was used for 60 years to relieve menopause symptoms until scientists discovered it increased breast cancer, heart disease, and stroke risk. Now, the hunt is on for safer alternatives, and researchers may have made a major discovery — a compound in soy that cuts hot flashes in half.

- Women going through menopause took 40 to 60 milligrams (mg) of daidzein, an isoflavone and phytoestrogen in soy, every day. After 12 weeks, they were suffering from half as many hot flashes as before, and the episodes were less severe.

- A Brazilian study had similar results. Forty women took 100 mg of soy isoflavones daily for 10 months and slashed the severity of their hot flashes by 70 percent, plus reduced the frequency.

You can easily get the same amount of daidzein, as well as total isoflavones, from eating half a cup of soybeans, one cup of soy milk, and an ounce of roasted soy nuts every day. Still, not all studies show soy helps menopause symptoms, which has left experts scratching their heads about what to tell women.

Daidzein is probably the compound responsible for improving symptoms in these studies. When you digest daidzein, the bacteria in your gut turn it into another compound, called equol. Not all women can produce equol equally. Some produce more than others. For instance, Asian women tend to produce more equol than Caucasian women. These digestive differences may explain why soy foods improve menopause symptoms in some women but not others.

In fact, a new study seems to prove just that. In women who could not make equol, soy supplements had no effect on menopause symptoms. But in women who could produce equol, soy improved hot flashes, sweating, weakness, heart palpitations, and tingling limbs.

Experts say you should have your equol levels tested before you take soy for menopausal symptoms. Ask your doctor how. And remember, the relief won't be as great as with estrogen replacement therapy, because the phytoestrogens in soy foods are simply not as strong as estrogen.

Straight talk about soy and memory loss

The link between soy and memory loss just became more worrisome. Earlier research found that people who ate soy foods more than twice a week had a higher risk of dementia and worse brain function with age. A new study backs up those findings. Seniors living on the island of Java who ate the most tofu had the worst memories.

That's not a complete surprise, since estrogen seems to increase the risk of dementia in women over age 65, and soy contains plant estrogens. Still, experts think both estrogens and phytoestrogens in foods, like soy, have a positive effect on your brain during youth and middle-age, then begin to do harm around age 65.

Tofu, tempeh, and miso aren't the only foods made from soybeans. Manufacturers add soy protein to breads, baked goods, hot cereals, pastas, whipped toppings, processed meats, and more to improve their texture and boost protein levels. Look for soy in the Ingredients list.

Another soy food, tempeh, seemed to offset some of the negative effects of tofu in the Java study. In fact, tempeh-lovers boasted better memories. This soy food contains more of the isoflavone genistein than tofu, as well as more folate because it is fermented. In fact, tempeh packs five times more folate than boiled soybeans, which are used to make tofu. Folate, in turn, may protect aging brains and reduce the risk of dementia.

The bottom line — as usual, too much of a good thing can be bad. The same goes for soy.

- Eat soy foods only in moderation.

- Consider trading in tofu for tempeh.

- Eat plenty of fruits, which were also linked to better memory in Java seniors.

- Talk to your doctor if you are concerned about soy's effects on your memory or brain function.

Easy Chocolate Mousse

Ingredients

3.5 oz chocolate instant pudding mix, small box

1 1/4 cups soy milk

10.5 oz tofu, silken

Instructions

1. Blend the chocolate pudding mix and the soy milk on medium speed for about 15 seconds until the mixture is very smooth.

2. Add the silken tofu and blend again. Scrape the mixture down off the sides. Blend and scrape until well mixed and very smooth.

3. Pour mixture into four small serving dishes.

4. Place in the refrigerator. Chill for at least two hours before serving.

(Serves 4)

Nutrition Summary by Serving

120.1 Calories (49.5 calories from fat, 41.18 percent of total); 5.5 g Fats; 8.9 g Protein; 10.5 g Carbohydrates; 1.5 mg Cholesterol; 1.3 g Fiber; 84.8 mg Sodium

Tomatoes

A double dose of heart protection

High blood pressure? You can get help from an amazing vegetable
that cleans arteries like a scrub brush. That's right. A tasty tomato can
help you fight high blood pressure and cholesterol at the same time.
But wait, isn't the tomato a fruit? Botanists call it a fruit, but chefs
and the U.S. Department of Agriculture call it a vegetable.
Fortunately, you can just call it heart smart.

Controls your blood pressure. People with mild high blood pressure
who took tomato extract lowered their systolic blood pressure by 10
points and their diastolic blood pressure by 4 points in just two months,
say researchers from Israel's University of the Negev. And the tomato
extract they took was equal to only a half cup of pasta sauce a day.

Participants also experienced less oxidation of their LDL cholesterol.
That's important because LDL cholesterol becomes far more dangerous
if it gets oxidized. Oxidation happens when molecules called free
radicals attack and damage LDL cholesterol. That triggers a process that
helps cholesterol turn into plaque on the inside of your arteries. As more
cholesterol gets oxidized, the plaque grows thicker and thicker, so it
hardens your arteries and narrows the space blood can pass through.
This contributes to high blood pressure and puts you at higher risk for a
heart attack. On top of that, oxidized LDL lowers the levels of nitric
oxide in your blood vessels. You need nitric oxide to help your blood
vessel walls stay flexible and open.

Scrubs your arteries clean. People who ate fresh tomatoes — or
drank tomato juice — not only lowered their LDL cholesterol, but
also raised their "good" HDL cholesterol in a study from Taiwan.
Some experts think HDL cholesterol can scrub cholesterol from the

plaque that's trying to block your arteries. That may prevent the hardening and narrowing of your arteries that contributes to your risk of high blood pressure and heart attack. So the more HDL you have, the better off you may be.

Lycopene — a natural antioxidant in tomatoes — may be the main trigger for all these heart-protecting effects, but other tomato nutrients like beta carotene and vitamin E may help as well. So add more tomatoes and tomato products to your diet. Since cooked tomatoes have more lycopene, be sure to enjoy treats like pasta sauce, ketchup, tomato soup, and tomato juice. Eat them with a little fat like olive oil so your body can absorb as much of their health-building lycopene as possible.

When you should never eat soup

Never eat soup from a grocery store or restaurant without checking the sodium content — especially if you have high blood pressure. Many are full of hidden salt and sugars. In fact, just one can of tomato soup made with milk has almost as much salt as five slices of bacon and more sugar than a blueberry muffin. So make your own healthy alternative instead. Start by puréeing 1/2 pound of fresh, peeled tomatoes. Not only do they taste fabulous, but they contain only about 10 mg of natural sodium. Heat them with either water or low-fat milk, and add delicious spices like thyme, curry powder, garlic, and fresh basil.

Delicious secret to smoother skin

Eating your favorite Italian dishes could be your ticket to preventing wrinkles, avoiding sunburn, and stopping skin cancer before it starts. You might even push back your skin's aging process.

According to scientists from two British universities, people who ate five tablespoons of tomato paste with a little olive oil each day showed 33 percent more resistance to sunburn. Even better, this "tomato diet" may also have anti-aging effects.

"The tomato diet boosted the level of procollagen in the skin significantly. These increasing levels suggest potential reversal of the skin aging process," says Professor Lesley Rhodes, a dermatologist at the University of Manchester. Procollagen is a molecule that helps your skin keep its proper structure. Low levels of procollagen reduce the suppleness of your skin and lead to aging — so the more you get, the better. What's more, Newcastle University researchers say the tomato diet may also reduce another possible cause of skin aging — the sun's ability to damage DNA in the mitochondria, those tiny power plants that produce energy in your cells.

Lycopene may be the secret behind tomato paste's success, the scientists say. When the sun damages your skin, that creates free-radical molecules. If too many free radicals are born, they can turn into a sort of demolition team that injures your skin's structure and opens the door for premature wrinkles and skin cancer. But lycopene is an antioxidant — the natural enemy and antidote to free radicals. That's why adding it to your diet may help defend your skin.

Just remember, the protective power of tomatoes isn't enough to replace your SPF 15 sunscreen. Instead, think of lycopene as your anti-aging sunscreen booster. To match the people in the study, aim for five tablespoons of tomato paste each day. Try adding it to pasta and pizza sauce, shrimp marinara, gumbo, chili, and more. It could be the yummiest way ever to younger-looking, cancer-free skin.

Hit the 'sauce' for stronger bones

Make marinara sauce, barbecue sauce, salsa, and even ketchup part of your daily diet, and you'll help keep brittle bones at bay.

University of Toronto scientists studied the food intake and tested the blood of 33 women between ages 50 and 60. They discovered that women who ate the most lycopene not only boosted the lycopene in their blood, but also had lower blood levels of a compound associated with bone loss. This is important because your skeleton is constantly getting rid of tired old bone and replacing it with new bone cells.

Unfortunately, as you get older, you start losing more bone than you add. That's why it's important to slow down "bone resorption" — your body's process for getting rid of old bone. According to the Canadian scientists, lycopene may help you do that.

Top lycopene eaters in the study only needed two tablespoons of tomato sauce or ketchup a day to see results, so why not give it a try? You'll enjoy delicious foods like tomato soup, pizza sauce, and Italian dishes. You can even add cheese for extra calcium as well as olive oil to make sure your body absorbs as much bone-saving lycopene as possible.

New weapon against prostate cancer

Good news for anyone who loves sun-dried tomatoes. A little-known compound in dried tomatoes may help prevent prostate cancer. What's more, it may make lycopene more effective at fighting this cancer.

University of Missouri scientists first uncovered this new cancer fighter in a test-tube study. They found that an amino acid called FruHis protected against the kind of DNA damage that leads to prostate cancer. But that's not all. When combined with lycopene, FruHis stopped cancer cell growth nearly every time.

But what happens in test tubes doesn't always work in live subjects, and the test-tube study used a concentrated form of FruHis. So scientists tested FruHis in animals. They fed some of the animals dried tomatoes or tomato paste made from dried tomatoes and also fed some of the animals extra FruHis. In the end, animals whose diet included tomato paste plus FruHis survived prostate cancer the longest. But even animals given tomato powder or tomato paste survived longer than animals on a standard diet.

The scientists say it's too early to tell whether eating sun-dried tomatoes or a dried-tomato paste can have the same positive effects on people, but you've got nothing to lose by giving it a try. Besides, sun-dried tomatoes are a delicious addition to almost any Italian dish you can think of. Add them in their regular dried form, or purée them. If you use a store-bought tomato paste, make sure the label says the paste contains sun-dried tomatoes for more prostate protection.

Special tomato packs more antioxidant punch

You've been told "redder is better" when it comes to lycopene. But an upstart orange tomato may turn that notion on its head.

According to Ohio State University scientists, people absorbed two-and-a-half times more lycopene from a sauce made from orange-colored tangerine tomatoes than from red tomato sauce. Apparently it has to do with the type of lycopene it contains. Red tomatoes are bursting with trans-lycopene, but another form called cis-lycopene is far easier for your body to absorb. Tangerine tomatoes are rich in this cis-lycopene, and your body pulls in those riches like a vacuum cleaner.

More studies are needed to see if cis-lycopene has the same health benefits as trans-lycopene. But if you're looking for a new tomato to grow in your garden, keep an eye out for tangerine tomatoes in your favorite nursery or seed catalog. You might be among the first to find out just how beneficial cis-lycopene can be.

Vinegar

Tasty way to tame blood sugar

A bedtime snack of cheese and vinegar could mean lower blood sugar in the morning, and a little vinegar with your food may lower blood sugar after a meal. Some experts even think vinegar works the same way as diabetes drugs.

Lower your a.m. blood sugar. People with diabetes had lower morning blood sugar readings when they ate two tablespoons of vinegar and an ounce of cheese right before bed, a small study from Arizona State University found. In fact, the readings were 6 percent lower for those who normally had the highest morning blood sugar readings. But the scientists think vinegar may team up with the protein in cheese to help keep your liver from producing too much blood sugar.

Avoid sugar spikes. Vinegar may pack even more power against the blood sugar spikes that follow a high-carb meal. And one study suggests it may be particularly effective if you have prediabetes or a high risk of diabetes. Before eating breakfast, 11 people with prediabetes and 10 with full-blown diabetes drank four teaspoons of apple cider vinegar in saccharin-sweetened water. A week later, they ate the same breakfast without the vinegar. Drinking vinegar cut after-breakfast blood sugar levels by nearly 20 percent for people with diabetes. Even better, it slashed blood sugar levels by 34 percent for people with prediabetes.

Experts suspect vinegar may block an enzyme your body normally uses to digest starches — the carbs that trigger blood sugar spikes. As a result, your body treats carbohydrates as waste instead of food, so they're swept out of your body when you visit the bathroom. The prescription medicine acarbose works the same way, say scientists behind the study. They point out that medicines like acarbose may reduce your odds of getting full-blown diabetes if you have prediabetes.

Balsamic vinegar, white vinegar, red wine vinegar, and apple cider vinegar may all work to cut after-meal blood sugar. If you'd like to give one a try, make sure the label on the bottle promises 5 percent acetic acid, and include it in salad dressings, marinades, soups, and sauces.

Keep pain pills in the cabinet

Nearly 22 percent of those with arthritis, fibromyalgia, or a similar condition said that vinegar helped their symptoms, an Indiana University survey reported. No studies have determined whether apple cider vinegar can help osteoarthritis symptoms, but some people swear by it. If you'd like to try this, mix one teaspoon of apple cider vinegar and one teaspoon of honey into a glass of water and drink every day. Be patient. Even enthusiasts admit that this remedy may take up to 12 months to ease your arthritis pain.

Add flavor and subtract cancer risk

You may have heard that cooking meats on the grill can raise your risk of cancer, but a little added seasoning means you can have your meat and heat it, too.

Beware of HCAs. When you cook meats on the grill, the high temperatures trigger chemical changes in the meat. As a result, cancer-causing heterocyclic amines (HCAs) start popping up like bubbles in boiling water. But marinating meats before grilling may squelch HCAs. A California study found that marinated chicken contained 92 to 99 percent fewer HCAs than unmarinated chicken.

Create a cancer barrier. Scientists think marinating creates a barrier against the high heat of grilling — like sitting in the shade instead of in the sun. You still get enough heat to cook your meat, but you end up with far fewer HCAs. Scientists aren't sure which marinade ingredients are behind this protection, but they suspect vinegar may be one of your key defenders.

The scientists in the study used a delicious marinade featuring apple cider vinegar, olive oil, garlic, lemon juice, mustard, brown sugar, and salt. They later discovered that brown sugar increased a certain type of HCA, but the rest of the ingredients cut HCAs as long as grilling lasted 30 minutes or less. So the next time you're getting ready for a cookout, make or buy a vinegar-based marinade and remember these tips.

- The kind of marinade you use is up to you, but the American Institute of Cancer Research recommends you include at least three key ingredients — an acid like vinegar, a base such as honey or oil, and a flavoring like garlic or onion.

- If you plan to use marinade as a sauce while grilling, separate it from the sauce you'll use for marinating before the marinating begins. Reusing marinade can contaminate perfectly good meat and may cause food poisoning.

- Marinate meat up to 24 hours to tenderize it as well as season it. But only marinate fish for 30 minutes or less or you'll end up with mush.

- Marinate meat in glass or in thick plastic food storage bags. Containers made of other substances may react with the vinegar.

Vinegar Dressing for Cole Slaw

Ingredients

1/2 cup sugar

1/2 cup apple cider vinegar

1/2 cup canola oil

1 tsp salt

1/2 tsp pepper

1/2 tsp celery seed

Instructions

1. Combine sugar, vinegar, and oil in a small saucepan. Heat to boiling.

2. Remove from heat, and add salt, pepper, and celery seed. Immediately pour over approximately 5 cups of shredded cabbage and other vegetables.

(Serves 8)

Nutrition Summary by Serving

173.2 Calories (123.0 calories from fat, 70.99 percent of total); 13.7 g Fats; 0.0 g Protein; 12.9 g Carbohydrates; 0.0 mg Cholesterol; 0.1 g Fiber; 295.7 mg Sodium

Fight your odds of a heart attack

Someday doctors may recommend vinegar as a healthy part of a heart-smart diet. Early studies suggest it may help you control your cholesterol and blood pressure.

A recent study found that animals who ate a high-cholesterol diet with added vinegar had lower cholesterol readings than animals who ate the high-cholesterol diet alone. Although scientists working for a corporate vinegar producer performed the study, other scientists considered it noteworthy enough to be published in the *British Journal of Nutrition*. The study suggests that vinegar may help fight cholesterol in two ways.

- It may trim your liver's ability to produce cholesterol.

- It may stimulate the removal of cholesterol-laden bile acid from your body.

An earlier study by the same vinegar producer suggested that rats prone to high blood pressure had lowered their readings by eating a diet with rice vinegar. The scientists behind that study think vinegar may help block renin, an enzyme that helps cause high blood pressure.

Of course, animals process foods differently than people, so more research is needed before scientists can recommend vinegar as a heart helper. But if you want to add more vinegar to your diet, try eating vinegar-based salad dressings in place of high-fat dressings. You can also add vinegar to soups or use it in place of high-fat seasonings recommended for your favorite recipes and dishes. Just avoid drinking it "straight" since vinegar can damage tooth enamel.

Clean house without harmful chemicals

Cut through grease and germs. Stop bacteria and mold. Even remove clothing stains and beat bathtub film. This inexpensive pantry classic is all you need. Here's how to clean your house from top to bottom with vinegar.

Freshen up the toilet bowl. A self-cleaning toilet bowl? You heard it right. This simple formula makes any toilet automatically spic and span. Pour in one cup of undiluted white vinegar. Let stand for five minutes. Flush. To fight germs, let the vinegar set overnight before flushing. To simply deodorize, pour in 3 cups of white vinegar, wait 30 minutes, and then flush.

Eliminate tub and tile film. Just wipe the surface with white vinegar, follow up with baking soda, and rinse with water. If you're out of baking soda, just use the vinegar and rinse.

Get shower curtains squeaky clean. Strip soap film, mildew, and grime off your shower curtains the easy way. Toss your curtains into the washing machine with a bath towel. Add 8 ounces of white vinegar during the rinse cycle. Dry on low for three minutes.

Shine stainless steel and clean chrome. Smooth smudges and dirt off your stainless steel appliances and your chrome, stainless steel, and ceramic fixtures. Dampen a sponge or soft cloth with white vinegar and wipe. Vinegar can be more powerful than you expect, so test this in an inconspicuous place first.

Make furniture gleam and glass rings vanish. Mix equal parts of white vinegar and vegetable oil together to make an all-natural furniture polish. White vinegar with olive oil works well — especially if you need to wipe up water rings made by damp glasses. Apply with a soft cloth and buff it off.

Turn windows streakless. Eliminate streaks and dirt from your windows with vinegar in a spray bottle. Dry with a soft cloth.

Erase cola and wine stains. Make these stains disappear from cotton, polyester, and permanent press cotton fabrics. For best results, do this within 24 hours. Sponge white vinegar on the stain and rub clean. Wash and dry as directed on the manufacturer's care tag.

Wipe deodorant stains away. Rub deodorant or antiperspirant stains lightly with white vinegar, wipe with a cloth, and then launder.

Remove stuck-on food from pots. Pour white vinegar into grimy, food-stained pots and pans and let soak for 30 minutes. Rinse with hot, soapy water. Vinegar is such a good grease cutter that some college cafeterias use it to clean fry vats and grill hoods.

Prevent mold and bacteria on counters. Wipe your counter tops with a vinegar-soaked cloth. The acid in vinegar cuts through the grease and germs on your counter tops. It has also been known to help fight bacteria and mold.

Melt away hard water deposits. Get both hard-water buildup and corrosion off your faucets and fixtures. Soak a paper towel in vinegar, wrap it around the faucet or fixture, and leave overnight. When morning comes, just wipe clean.

Household Hint

Simple cure for clogged drains

Put away the plunger. Vinegar can open your clogged drain and get rid of odors, too. Heat one cup of vinegar, pour a cup of baking soda down the drain, and follow it with the heated vinegar. The resulting fizz will create a chemical reaction that breaks down the fatty acids in a greasy clog. That makes the clog easier to shatter and scatter. After 15 minutes, just pour a quart of water down the drain and flush the clog away.

If the clog is particularly stubborn, don't worry. Just try a second time, or leave the mixture to cook overnight before rinsing. It's cheaper than a plumber or chemicals, and you won't wear out your arms trying to use the plunger.

Meet your indoor-outdoor problem solver

Make your life easier both inside the house and out. Just look at all the ways vinegar can help you.

- Don't pay ridiculous prices for age-spot creams. Make your own with two ingredients from your kitchen. Just combine vinegar with an equal amount of onion juice, and dab this all-natural remedy on age spots daily. You should start seeing results in a few weeks.

- Easily remove salt stains or buildup from clay and plastic flower pots. Just fill the kitchen sink with two parts cold water and one part white vinegar. Soak the pots and their saucers until they look stain-free, and then wash with soap and water.

- Keep cheese fresher and mold-free longer. Dampen a paper towel with apple cider vinegar, wrap it around the cheese, and drop the wrapped cheese into a sealable food storage bag. Keep in the fridge. You may be surprised at how long it will last.

- Loosen rusty spigots, screws, nuts, and bolts by soaking them in vinegar.

- Forget those expensive fruit and veggie washes. Instead, soak your produce in vinegar for 15 minutes to remove dirt, pesticides, and wax. But don't try this on fruit with little pores or hairs. They'll end up tasting funny.

- Keep rabbits from eating your plants. After you empty a spice dispenser or salt shaker, soak a cotton ball with vinegar and drop it in. Put the hole-covered top back on, and leave it near the plants you want to protect.

- Make a light and flaky pie crust. Add a teaspoon of vinegar to the cold water used to make the dough.

- Lime in the garden may make your plants thrive, but it can leave your hands rough, flaky, and drier than the Sahara desert. Soothe them by rinsing your hands in white vinegar right after using lime. You'll love how much better your hands feel.

- Vinegar can do double duty at your hummingbird feeder. Use it to clean your feeder, and you'll avoid the chemical residue soaps and detergents can leave behind. But don't put the bottle away when you're done. If wasps have been stealing your hummer's food, just soak a cotton ball in vinegar and place it near the feeder.

- Acid-loving plants like azaleas, rhododendrons, gardenias, and mountain laurels may not do as well if you have hard water, so make them an "energy drink." Mix one cup of vinegar into one gallon of water and pour it around the base of your plants. Not only will your plants get the acid environment they love, but this also helps them draw iron from the soil.

Household Hint

Conquer ants the easy way

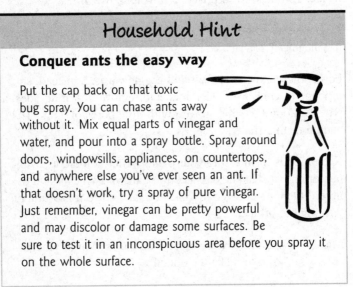

Put the cap back on that toxic bug spray. You can chase ants away without it. Mix equal parts of vinegar and water, and pour into a spray bottle. Spray around doors, windowsills, appliances, on countertops, and anywhere else you've ever seen an ant. If that doesn't work, try a spray of pure vinegar. Just remember, vinegar can be pretty powerful and may discolor or damage some surfaces. Be sure to test it in an inconspicuous area before you spray it on the whole surface.

Vitamin D

Sunshine vitamin shields you from cancer

Inga from Norway is five times more likely to get ovarian cancer than her friend Carmen in Brazil. And attorney Ted is more likely to develop prostate cancer than his cousin Fred, who works construction. What's the difference? Carmen and Fred get a lot more vitamin D — the sunshine vitamin that could hold the key to cancer prevention.

Vitamin D, which your body produces when exposed to the sun's ultraviolet rays, is found naturally in fatty fish and in fortified foods, like milk and cereal. You can also take a multivitamin or vitamin D supplement to boost your levels. No matter how you get your vitamin D, you probably should get more of it. Low levels of vitamin D or sun exposure have been linked to a variety of cancers — and boosting your intake may boost your defense.

Super sources of vitamin D

* fortified milk
* fortified cereal
* salmon
* cheese
* tuna
* liver
* mackerel
* egg yolks

A recent study of older women found that those who took vitamin D and calcium supplements had a 60 percent lower risk for all cancers. That makes sense, considering at least 200 human genes respond to vitamin D. Many of these genes play a role in helping to regulate the multiplying and death of cells — key processes in cancer development.

Here's a look at some specific cancers and the evidence that supports vitamin D's role in fighting them.

Breast. A Harvard study found that women with the highest blood levels of vitamin D had lower risks of breast cancer — but only if the women were over age 60. Conversely, another Harvard study found that women who get a lot of vitamin D and calcium cut their risk of breast cancer by almost one-third, but the link was only found in women who have not yet gone through menopause.

A recent study estimates that 350,000 cases of breast cancer worldwide could be prevented just by boosting vitamin D intakes. And pooled data for 980 women show a 50 percent lower risk of breast cancer for those with the highest intake compared to those with the lowest. Lab studies show that vitamin D can treat large breast tumors by boosting apoptosis, or cell death, and slowing down the spread of tumor cells.

Colon. A Harvard study found a lower risk for colon cancer for women over age 60 with higher blood levels of vitamin D. A Korean study of U.S. women found that higher intakes of vitamin D led to a lower risk of colon cancer. In a University of Hawaii study, an increased intake of vitamin D lowered the risk for men, but not for women. Researchers estimate that 250,000 cases of colon cancer worldwide may be prevented by boosting vitamin D intakes.

Lung. Lack of sunlight may boost your risk of lung cancer, according to a recent study of cancer rates in over 100 countries. Researchers say vitamin D, which can halt tumor growth by promoting cell death, could be the reason that sunlight helps.

Ovarian. The risk of ovarian cancer is five times higher for women living in high latitudes, like Norway and Iceland, compared to those living in countries near the equator, where you get more sunlight.

Pancreatic. In a recent study of 46,000 men and 75,000 women, those who got at least 600 International Units (IU) of vitamin D each day had a 40 percent lower risk of pancreatic cancer than those who got less than 150 IU a day.

Prostate. In a study of men with prostate cancer, the cancer developed three to five years later in those who worked outdoors rather than indoors. Prostate tissue, like breast and colon tissue, produces vitamin D locally to keep cell growth in check. More sun means more vitamin D — and less out-of-control cell growth.

While protecting yourself from other cancers, you don't want to put yourself at increased risk for skin cancer from too much exposure to the sun. A combination of diet, supplements, and short periods of time — such as 10 to 15 minutes a day — in the sun without sunscreen should do the trick.

Ease chronic pain

Not getting enough vitamin D can be a real pain — literally. In a recent study, about one in four people suffering from chronic pain had a vitamin D deficiency. They also needed higher doses of morphine for a longer period of time to deal with the pain. That's because low levels of vitamin D can cause pain and muscle weakness, and these pain-related symptoms of vitamin D deficiency do not respond well to pain medications. The solution may be as simple as boosting your vitamin D intake with supplements.

Revive weak bones and muscles

The calcium in milk helps keep your bones strong, but milk comes with an added bonus — vitamin D. This key vitamin helps strengthen bones and muscles. It can also help reduce your risk of falling.

Osteoporosis, or brittle bone disease, can lead to broken hips, arms, or wrists. You may also have a stooped posture or lower back pain.

Women, especially, should take steps to guard against it. That's where vitamin D comes in.

First of all, vitamin D helps your body absorb calcium. If you don't get enough vitamin D, chances are you're not getting enough calcium, either. And you know how essential this mineral is for optimum bone health. With or without calcium, vitamin D helps boost the bone density of hips and other bones. The results of several studies showed that people who took 700 to 800 International Units (IU) of vitamin D a day had a 26 percent lower risk of hip fractures than people who took a placebo.

In addition to bones, vitamin D also makes muscles stronger. Muscle tissue has receptors specifically designed to accept vitamin D. When researchers gave vitamin D supplements to older women, it resulted in an increase in protein synthesis, which means an increase in muscle growth and size. Studies of older people found that those with higher levels of vitamin D perform better on tests that include walking and getting out of a chair.

Not surprisingly, considering its positive effect on bones and muscles, vitamin D may help improve your balance. In a recent Australian study, people taking vitamin D supplements lowered their risk of falls by 19 percent.

Surprising way to avoid arthritis

Advertisements trumpet supplements like glucosamine and chondroitin to treat osteoarthritis, the most common form of arthritis. But you may be able to protect your joints just by getting enough vitamin D. Studies revealed that arthritis of the knee and hip were more likely to develop in people with low levels of vitamin D. The reason could stem from this important vitamin's ability to protect the cartilage that cushions your joints. When cartilage wears away, it leaves your knees, hips, and other joints feeling stiff and sore.

As if that's not enough, vitamin D boosts the quality of your bones, reducing the risk of bone spurs that lead to arthritis pain. Not only does vitamin D help your bones, it also helps your body absorb calcium, a key bone-building mineral. Your body also needs vitamin D for normal cartilage metabolism.

Vitamin D may help you live longer. According to a recent analysis of 18 studies, people taking vitamin D supplements had a 7 percent lower risk of death from any cause.

Spend more time in the sunlight and drink more milk, and maybe you'll give your joints a fighting chance against osteoarthritis.

Take a bite out of tooth loss

You can guard your gums by boosting your intake of a powerful anti-inflammatory — vitamin D. Several studies show a link between low vitamin D levels and periodontal disease, the leading cause of tooth loss in older people.

Periodontal disease is caused by chronic inflammation, which leads to receding gums. In one study, older people who were given 700 International Units (IU) of vitamin D and 500 milligrams (mg) of calcium a day for three years had 60 percent less tooth loss than those who took a placebo. Vitamin D likely helps because it suppresses inflammation.

An early sign of periodontal disease is gingivitis, or gum disease. This painful condition features sore, irritated gums that bleed during brushing, flossing, and oral exams. In a recent study, people with the highest levels of vitamin D in their blood were 20 percent less likely to suffer from bleeding gums during an oral exam compared to those with the lowest blood levels. That's because the anti-inflammatory effects of vitamin D help limit gum irritation.

Besides taking supplements, you can add vitamin D to your diet by eating more salmon and fortified dairy products. Other steps you should take to protect your teeth and gums include brushing and flossing regularly and visiting your dentist every six months.

Surprisingly simple way to stay healthy

Gum disease is bad enough, but evidence suggests it can lead to even more serious problems. In a recent Harvard study of male doctors, those with a history of gum disease had a 64 percent higher risk of developing pancreatic cancer. Inflammation of the gums could trigger inflammation in the rest of your body, which contributes to cancer. Other studies have linked gum disease to heart disease, diabetes, and rheumatoid arthritis — and inflammation likely is to blame. Luckily, vitamin D helps stamp out inflammation, making it an effective weapon against gum disease — and all the risks that come with it.

Why your eyes need vitamin D

Got milk? If you want to protect your eyesight, your answer should be yes. The vitamin D in milk may help prevent age-related macular degeneration, or AMD. Age-related macular degeneration, the leading cause of blindness in older people, robs you of your central vision. You may see grayness, haziness, or a blank spot in the center of your field of vision. Words on a page may look blurry, straight lines may seem wavy or distorted, and colors may seem dimmer.

But getting more vitamin D can brighten your outlook. A recent study found that high blood levels of vitamin D meant a lower risk of early age-related macular degeneration. Compared to people with the lowest blood levels, those with the highest levels reduced their risk by 36 percent.

Researchers also looked at some common food sources of vitamin D — milk and fish. Drinking milk reduced the risk for early AMD by 25 percent, while eating fish lowered the risk of advanced AMD by 59 percent. Vitamin D supplements also helped — but only for those who didn't drink milk daily. In those cases, supplements cut the risk of early AMD by one-third.

Vitamin D likely fights AMD because of its anti-inflammatory powers. Laboratory and population studies link inflammation to AMD — and vitamin D has been shown to decrease the production of inflammatory cells.

Slam the brakes on autoimmune disorders

When your immune system turns on you, turn to vitamin D. Higher levels of this key vitamin may help you avoid autoimmune disorders, such as multiple sclerosis, rheumatoid arthritis, and Crohn's disease. All three of these conditions occur more often the further you go from the equator, where people get less sun exposure — which means less vitamin D production. But that's not the only evidence that vitamin D plays a key role in their prevention.

Researchers found that women who took at least 400 International Units (IU) of vitamin D daily had a 40 percent lower risk of developing multiple sclerosis (MS). In a study of military personnel, those with the highest blood levels of vitamin D were 62 percent less likely to develop MS compared to those with the lowest levels.

Vitamin D levels are often low in people with rheumatoid arthritis, a condition where your immune system attacks your joints. Some studies of mice had success suppressing or preventing autoimmune diseases, including rheumatoid arthritis, inflammatory bowel disease — which includes Crohn's disease — and type 1 diabetes.

That's probably because of vitamin D's effect on your immune response, especially macrophages and T-cells. Vitamin D decreases the production of T-1 helper cells, the kind that attack your body in autoimmune diseases, and boosts the formation of T-2 helper cells. Vitamin D and macrophages also work together to put a damper on an overactive immune system. When you don't get enough vitamin D, your immune system can spiral out of control, which is what happens in autoimmune disorders. Boosting your vitamin D levels, by spending more time in the sun, taking supplements, or eating more fortified foods, may boost your defense against your own immune system.

Household Hint

Smart supplement strategies

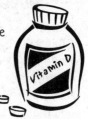

Shopping for vitamin D supplements can be tricky. You'll find two types — vitamin D2 and vitamin D3. While both will give you some benefit, opt for vitamin D3, or cholecalciferol, which is more potent and longer-acting.

How much vitamin D you should get depends on your age. Current guidelines call for 200 International Units (IU) a day up to age 50, 400 IU daily from age 51 to 70, and 600 IU daily after age 70. But many experts think these recommended amounts are too low. For example, if you're middle-age or older, they say aim for 1,000 IU daily. Just keep in mind that vitamin D can be toxic at extremely high doses, so don't go overboard.

Unusual strategy to stop weight gain

Your weight can be a heavy factor in conditions like heart disease and diabetes. If you're a woman, taking vitamin D and calcium supplements may help you keep off those extra pounds after you reach menopause. In a seven-year study of more than 36,000 women ages 50 to 79, those who took the supplements gained less weight than those who did not. The overall effect was small — an average of less than a half pound — but it was greater among women who weren't getting enough calcium at the start of the study. Vitamin D and calcium may stimulate the breakdown of fat cells and block the development of new ones.

Breathe better with vitamin D

Here's some news that might make you breathe a sigh of relief. Vitamin D can give your lungs a boost if you're struggling with asthma or other breathing problems. Blood levels of vitamin D may have an impact on lung function. New Zealand researchers measured forced expiratory volume (FEV), or how much air you can exhale in one second, and forced vital capacity (FVC), the amount you can blow after a deep breath when exhaling as rapidly as possible.

People with the highest vitamin D levels also had stronger FEV and FVC scores. The link was strongest in people older than age 60. Vitamin D may help by remodeling tissues in your lungs. While it's still too early to know for sure, raising your vitamin D intake could help with respiratory conditions like chronic obstructive pulmonary disease (COPD), asthma, and emphysema.

Actually, vitamin D supplements can help treat asthma. Some people with asthma do not respond to steroid treatment. But researchers from

King's College in London found that vitamin D3 supplements can help these people. Steroids work by spurring your immune system's T-cells to produce a signaling molecule called IL-10 that blocks the immune response that causes asthma symptoms.

The T-cells of nonresponders do not produce IL-10 — but they do when vitamin D3 supplements are added to the mix. As a bonus, the supplements can even help healthy people or those who already respond to steroids by making their T-cells more responsive to steroids. Taking vitamin D supplements could be an easy, effective way to control your asthma and enjoy a breath of fresh air.

Heart disease self-defense

High blood pressure and high cholesterol put you at high risk for heart problems. On the other hand, a high intake of vitamin D may offer some protection. A recent New Zealand study of a cross-section of the United States population found a link between vitamin D and blood pressure. People with higher blood levels of vitamin D had lower blood pressure. This link, which was stronger for people age 50 and older, helps explain why blood pressure is often higher in black people than white people. People with darker skin produce less vitamin D than those with lighter skin. Boosting your vitamin D intake, by spending more time in the sun or taking supplements, may help lower your blood pressure.

Vitamin D supplements also helped dieting women further lower their cholesterol levels in another recent study. Losing weight has a beneficial effect on cholesterol, but women taking calcium and vitamin D supplements had much greater reductions in LDL cholesterol, as well as the ratios of total cholesterol to LDL cholesterol and LDL to HDL cholesterol. These healthy changes in cholesterol happened regardless of how much weight the women lost or how much their waist sizes changed.

Researchers suspect calcium helps block fat absorption, burn fat, and control your appetite — and your body needs vitamin D to absorb calcium. They also suggest that overweight women who do not get enough calcium or vitamin D should consider taking supplements to lower their risk of heart disease.

Dodge diabetes with a vital vitamin

Low levels of vitamin D could mean a higher risk for diabetes. In an Italian study, people with diabetes were much more likely to have a vitamin D deficiency. Women, people with poorly controlled diabetes, and those taking insulin or cholesterol-lowering drugs were even more likely to be deficient in this key vitamin. Another study found that people with the highest levels of vitamin D have a 75 percent lower risk of diabetes than those with the lowest levels — but researchers are not sure if vitamin D levels are a cause or an effect of diabetes.

Vitamin D supplements may help slow the progression of diabetes. In a study of older people with pre-diabetes — a condition marked by high blood sugar but not yet officially diabetes — those who took vitamin D and calcium supplements saw their blood sugar go up much less over the next three years than those who took a placebo. A Harvard study of 84,000 nurses found that those who supplemented their diet with at least 1,200 milligrams (mg) of calcium and 800 International Units (IU) of vitamin D cut their diabetes risk by one-third.

While it's not entirely clear how vitamin D helps with diabetes, it may promote insulin secretion from the beta islet cells in your pancreas. It may also influence insulin resistance. Many people with diabetes are overweight, which increases your need for vitamin D. As a fat-soluble vitamin, vitamin D is stored in fat cells, leaving less in the bloodstream. That makes it even more important to get additional vitamin D if you're overweight.

Besides diet and supplements, you can get vitamin D by spending more time in the sun. Ten to 15 minutes every day is a safe way to boost vitamin D levels without putting yourself at higher risk for skin cancer.

Vitamin E

Guard your heart and blood vessels

Vitamin E may have fallen out of favor for preventing heart disease, but don't count it out just yet. Studies show this nutrient can still benefit your circulation and even help prevent heart attacks in people with diabetes.

Avoid heart attack and stroke. Roughly three out of every eight people with diabetes have a gene that makes them more likely to have heart problems than other people with diabetes — a whopping two to five times more likely, in fact.

The Hp gene makes an antioxidant that sweeps up free radicals floating around your body before they can damage cells. But people with a version of the gene called Hp 2-2 make less effective antioxidants. The result — people with Hp 2-2 who have diabetes suffer a lot more damage from free radicals and a dramatically higher risk of heart problems.

That's where vitamin E comes in. In a new study, people with diabetes who took 400 IU of vitamin E

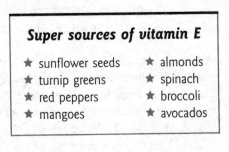

Super sources of vitamin E

- ★ sunflower seeds
- ★ turnip greens
- ★ red peppers
- ★ mangoes
- ★ almonds
- ★ spinach
- ★ broccoli
- ★ avocados

daily for 18 months slashed their risk of stroke, heart attack, and heart-related death in half, compared to people not on vitamin E.

Unfortunately, you can't get this much E from eating food, but piling your plate with foods rich in it won't hurt. Talk to your doctor before you try supplements, since vitamin E can increase the risk of death. According to the study researchers, only people with the Hp 2-2 gene should consider supplements.

Slice your risk of DVT. In deep vein thrombosis (DVT), a blood clot forms in the veins of your lower leg. Besides being painful, it's also dangerous, because the clot can break loose and travel to your lungs. This condition, pulmonary embolism, is the third most common cause of vascular death.

Women in a Harvard study significantly lowered their risk by upping their vitamin E intake. Out of nearly 40,000 women, those who had already suffered from venous thromboembolism, the condition that leads to DVT, sliced their risk of recurrence a whopping 44 percent. Other women cut their risk between 18 and 27 percent.

Conquer peripheral arterial disease (PAD). This disease occurs when the arteries in your legs or arms become clogged with fatty deposits, or plaques. They narrow and harden, restricting blood flow and nutrients to your hands and feet. Experts at the University of California found that out of more than 7,000 people, those who ate foods filled with vitamins E, C, A, and B6 as well as folate, fiber, and omega-3 fats were least likely to develop PAD.

Thank goodness for avocados, then. They're chock full of many of these nutrients, making them perfect for protecting your blood vessels. From fiber and folate to vitamins E, C, and K, they're a powerhouse food right on your produce aisle.

Dodge the common cold

Move over vitamin C and echinacea. Vitamin E is the latest weapon in the dirty war against colds and flu. You've probably already noticed your immune system tends to get weaker with age. This decline leaves you more susceptible to infections from viruses, bacteria, and other organisms.

Nearly every cell in your immune system changes as you get older, but T-cells change the most. Your body produces fewer T-cells with age, and those it does create don't work as well as they used to. Experts think this drop in T-cell function is the main reason the elderly have weaker immune systems.

Fortify your natural defenses. New research shows vitamin E could put the brakes on this decline and give your immune system a much-needed lift.

▪ T-cells need a substance called PGE-2 to work, but at high levels it actually stops T-cells from multiplying. Vitamin E steps in to keep PGE-2 from getting out of hand.

Skip supplements for longer life

You may be taking antioxidant supplements to lengthen your life, but research suggests they do just the opposite. A new review pooled the results of 67 studies. Taking supplements of vitamins A, E, or beta carotene increased, not decreased, people's risk of death.

One possible reason — when you get vitamin E and other antioxidants in food, you get normal, healthy amounts of them. In these small amounts, they act like antioxidants by protecting your cells. But in large amounts, research shows they actually do the opposite, causing oxidation and cell damage. This extra physical stress may hasten death.

The lesson — all good things in moderation. You're safe taking a regular multivitamin, but avoid megadoses of any nutrient.

- A certain molecule binds to T-cells and triggers them to mature and multiply. Unfortunately, your body produces less of this molecule with age, one major reason for T-cell decline. Vitamin E, however, boosts its production.

- Vitamin E also increases your levels of a molecule that kills invading viruses and delivers a shot in the arm to the whole virus-fighting network in your body.

Crush the common cold. Out of 600 seniors in a nursing home, those given 200 IU of vitamin E daily for one year developed fewer respiratory infections, including fewer cases of the common cold. Experts consider vitamin E one of the most effective nutrients for aiding your immune system, and it's easy to see why. Supplements can be dangerous, however, so focus on eating more foods rich in this cold-busting nutrient.

Ultimate vitamin adds vim and vigor

You are what you eat, and the older you get, the more your body notices. If you want to stay spry into your 80s, focus on eating a diet rich in vitamin E.

Your body needs certain nutrients, such as vitamin E, to repair itself. Without them, cells, muscles, joints, and other tissue breaks down. Seniors with low levels of this important vitamin were 62 percent more likely to lose physical function with age, an Italian study found.

As an antioxidant, vitamin E neutralizes free radicals that otherwise would damage cells and tissue through a process called oxidation. Free radicals are particularly dangerous to muscle and brain cells. Low levels of E are also linked to hardening of the arteries and brain disorders. These, in turn, can affect your mobility and physical function.

Exercising can help you stay active. Unfortunately, it also creates free radicals. So while it's important to keep fit, it's equally important to eat plenty of vitamin E in foods to offset the effects of exercise.

Researchers say vitamin E supplements won't necessarily prevent physical decline, but foods could. If you're trying to cut fat from your diet, however, you may be sabotaging your health. The best sources of vitamin E are often high in fat, such as olive oil, wheat germ, nuts, and seeds. Luckily, they're packed with good fats, such as poly- and monounsaturated fats, and not saturated or trans fats.

You don't need much vitamin E, either. Just getting 15 to 30 milligrams daily can raise your blood levels out of the danger zone linked to physical decline in the Italian study.

Weigh benefits of vitamin E for cancer

A new review shows that taking antioxidant supplements during chemotherapy reduced chemo side effects in 24 out of 33 studies. In some cases, people were able to withstand higher doses of chemo if they were on antioxidants.

Vitamin E supplements may help people receiving chemotherapy, but they can interfere with tamoxifen treatment. This drug blocks the activity of estrogen in breast tissue to help prevent the growth of breast cancer.

In five out of seven women, vitamin E supplements lowered the amount of tamoxifen in their system. What's more, estrogen was more active in breast cells in women taking vitamin E while on tamoxifen.

Super nutrient saves your hearing

Canola oil, avocado, wheat germ, and other rich sources of vitamin E could be just what you need to prevent hearing loss.

Loud noises produce free radicals inside your ear. These dangerous compounds trigger a process called oxidation, which can damage the delicate sensory cells in your ear that enable you to hear. Antioxidants like vitamin E come to the rescue by neutralizing free radicals before they permanently damage cells.

Antioxidants also keep the blood vessels that nourish those sensory cells from narrowing. When free radicals form, they create a by-product that constricts the blood vessels in your ear. This cuts the blood flow to those damaged hearing cells, so they can't heal effectively. By nixing free radicals, antioxidants keep those crucial blood vessels wide open and relaxed.

- Hearing improved 63 percent in people with sudden hearing loss who took a combination of vitamins C and E supplements and medication, compared to just 44 percent in people only taking medication.

- Giving guinea pigs a combination of antioxidant vitamins C, A, E, and magnesium just before exposing them to loud noise helped prevent hearing loss. Individual nutrients, however, didn't. The combination seemed to be key.

Researchers say you need to get these nutrients at least two days before being around loud noise in order to prevent hearing damage. But you can get ongoing protection by packing your plate with more olive oil for vitamin E, fruits for vitamin C, orange and red vegetables for beta carotene, and whole grains for magnesium. These nutrients may be able to reverse some hearing loss if taken within three days of noise exposure, but talk to your doctor before trying supplements.

Water & electrolytes

Top off your tank for better health

Water may be the cheapest anti-aging agent that does it all for your body. Everything from lips to kidneys can benefit from the powers of this vital part of your diet.

About two-thirds of your body is made of water, and it's important to keep nearly all your systems working properly. If you lose just a small percentage of your body's water, you can be dehydrated. That causes your blood volume to go down and sodium levels to go up. Then your fluid-regulating hormone levels change, and your kidneys slow down their job of making urine so you can conserve water. Finally, your brain lets you know you're thirsty, but it's a delayed message. That message may be even further delayed during cold weather.

Drink up — even before thirst hits — to benefit your body in these four ways.

- Prevent kidney stones. Without enough fluid to keep your kidneys working, crystals of calcium and uric acid can build up into painful kidney stones.

- Keep tissues moist. Your lips, eyes, and nose need water to stay hydrated.

- Head off head pain. Drinking too little is a common cause of headaches.

- Prevent constipation. Fiber keeps things moving, but you need water to help the fiber work.

Seniors are at special risk of dehydration, because they may not feel thirst as quickly as they did when they were younger. Residents of a senior home in England who made the effort to drink more water found they had more energy, were more alert, and felt happier.

Experts debate how much you should drink, but they usually suggest six or eight 8-ounce glasses a day — more in hot weather or during exercise. Don't forget you get water from foods like fruits and vegetables, which may be up to 90 percent water. And while you may have heard caffeinated drinks, like coffee and tea, don't count toward your fluid intake, they do. Any water-losing effect of the caffeine is offset by the water in these drinks. You can tell you're well hydrated if your urine looks the color of lemonade. If it's dark yellow or brown, you probably need to drink more.

Household Hint

Cheap way to banish grime

Cooking with less salt? Don't let that big, round, salt container go to waste. You can put that salt to good use cleaning a variety of items around your house.

- Sprinkle a little salt on brown paper, then run your hot iron over it to remove stickiness.

- Make a paste with salt and lemon juice, then carefully rub it on rusted scissors with a dry cloth. Rust comes off, scissors stay sharp.

- Put salt, crushed ice, and water in your glass coffee pot — just make sure the pot isn't hot. Swirl the mixture to remove stains, then rinse it out.

Indulge without guilt

Coconut milk, with its saturated fat and calories, has a bad reputation when it comes to health. But don't confuse coconut milk — creamy, white, and from mature coconuts — with coconut water — thinner, watery, and from young, green coconuts.

Coconut water is a naturally healthy drink. It's a good source of electrolytes, including calcium, magnesium, and potassium. In fact, one cup of coconut water has more potassium than a banana. The flavorful drink doesn't have any saturated fat, and it has less than 10 percent of the calories in the same amount of coconut milk. You can buy pasteurized coconut water in natural food stores.

3 great reasons to drink more water

Rev up your energy, curb your appetite, or increase the calories you're burning. Water will do all three depending on when you enjoy it. And it has zero calories — no matter how much you indulge.

Boost your energy. First thing when you wake up, you're bound to need a drink. That's because you tend to be dehydrated after a night's sleep, especially seniors. Classic signs of dehydration include fatigue, weakness, and feeling lightheaded. Get some water in your body to perk up your energy — without filling up on pancakes and bacon. A full glass of water — preferably 12 ounces — along with a healthy breakfast should do the trick.

Eat less. Drink some water before a meal to quiet your stomach rumblings. Then you won't feel the need to overeat during the meal. Researchers found that people who drank about two cups of water 30 minutes before lunch felt more full and didn't eat as much. You can also satisfy your hunger by eating fruits and vegetables because they have a high water content. The water fills you up, yet has no calories.

Burn more calories. You can charge up your body to burn more calories by drinking water throughout the day. That's because your metabolism — the rate your body burns calories — goes up about 10 minutes after you drink water. The metabolism boost is around 30 percent, and it lasts for more than an hour. So if you increase the amount of water you drink by about 1 1/2 quarts over the course of a day, you can burn about 48 calories more — all without lifting a finger.

Besides that, people who drink water tend to take in fewer calories during the day than people who drink other beverages. Stick with plain water, not one of the flavored fitness waters in a bottle. Some of these have almost as many calories as soda.

The latest scoop on low-salt diets

Common advice for people with high blood pressure or heart disease is to cut down on salt in their diets. Yet, new research shows this warning may be unhealthy for some people. The problem with salt is what it's made of — sodium and chloride. These two electrolytes work with water to help your cells function efficiently and keep your blood volume where it should be. Your doctor may urge you to limit your salt intake so these electrolytes stay in balance. Too much sodium can cause your body to hold onto water, increasing your blood volume and raising your blood pressure.

Then again, not everyone benefits from following a low-salt diet.

Limit your beverages if you suffer from an overactive bladder. If you have to "go" quite often — sometimes suddenly — you may have this condition. Cut down on what you drink by about a quarter, and your symptoms may improve. But don't reduce liquids too much — your body needs them to function.

Certain people are salt sensitive, which means their blood pressure reacts strongly when they eat salt. That's only about half the people who have high blood pressure, so experts are debating whether everyone should eat less salt. Following a low-salt diet causes other changes in your body, like making you more sensitive to insulin and changing how your sympathetic nervous system works. These changes may actually increase your risk of heart problems.

Unless you've been told you're salt-sensitive, your best advice may be to eat a healthy diet, keeping all electrolytes in balance — including sodium, magnesium, potassium, and calcium. And don't neglect the water needed to keep these minerals flowing. One study found drinking at least five glasses of water each day may lower your risk of dying from heart disease.

Experts say adults ages 19 to 50 — whether or not they have high blood pressure — should limit sodium intake to no more than 1,500 milligrams (mg) a day, or less than a teaspoon of salt. That can be pretty difficult to follow, considering how much sodium is hidden in processed foods. People older than age 50 are urged to limit sodium to 1,300 mg a day, while those over age 70 should limit sodium to 1,200 mg a day.

Flush out cancer risk

Water can do great things to keep your body running smoothly. Getting enough may also wash away deadly diseases, like cancer. The American Cancer Society urges you to drink water to reduce the risk of two types of cancer — bladder and colon.

A 10-year study found drinking about six 8-ounce glasses of water a day may reduce your risk of bladder cancer by 50 percent. It sounds simple, but it works because water flushes out carcinogens — cancer-causing substances in your urinary tract.

A similar action is at work when it comes to water and colon cancer — the third-most common type of cancer in the United States. Experts say changing what people eat could cut colon cancer deaths by 90 percent. Researchers in Seattle found that middle-age people who drank at least five glasses of water every day had the least risk of developing colon cancer. Water seems to dilute carcinogens in your bowels and flush them out more quickly. Other healthy foods that seem to ward off the disease include fruits and vegetables, hot and cold cereals, and dairy products.

And you don't need to spend a lot of money buying special water. You can stick with good-old tap water, which costs less than a penny a gallon. Bottled water costs about a thousand times more.

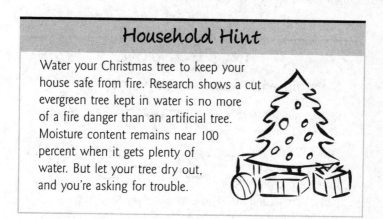

Household Hint

Water your Christmas tree to keep your house safe from fire. Research shows a cut evergreen tree kept in water is no more of a fire danger than an artificial tree. Moisture content remains near 100 percent when it gets plenty of water. But let your tree dry out, and you're asking for trouble.

Outsmart tooth decay

About two-thirds of Americans live in cities with fluoridated water. There's been much controversy over adding fluoride to public water, but half a century of research shows it can help strengthen teeth and prevent cavities. In fact, the U.S. Centers for Disease Control and Prevention estimates drinking fluoridated water cuts your rate of tooth decay by up to 40 percent.

A new study shows seniors can benefit from drinking fluoridated water even more than kids. Researchers looked at health records of children, adults, and seniors living in places with or without fluoride in the water. Everyone in the study had dental insurance, but there were differences in how much money was spent filling cavities and doing other procedures. Generally, people with fluoride in their water had lower dental costs, and seniors benefited more than children.

Fluoride works by binding to calcium, sodium, and other positively charged ions. That means it's attracted to calcium in teeth and bones, where it helps make them stronger. Fluoride is especially helpful for older people with gingivitis, since it helps mineralize exposed surfaces of tooth roots. Scientists are also working to see if fluoride can help strengthen bones to stop osteoporosis.

Household Hint

Save big with waterless car wash

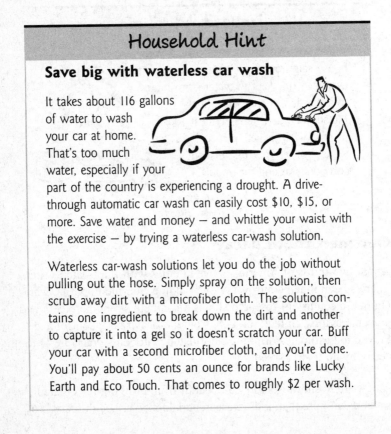

It takes about 116 gallons of water to wash your car at home. That's too much water, especially if your part of the country is experiencing a drought. A drive-through automatic car wash can easily cost $10, $15, or more. Save water and money — and whittle your waist with the exercise — by trying a waterless car-wash solution.

Waterless car-wash solutions let you do the job without pulling out the hose. Simply spray on the solution, then scrub away dirt with a microfiber cloth. The solution contains one ingredient to break down the dirt and another to capture it into a gel so it doesn't scratch your car. Buff your car with a second microfiber cloth, and you're done. You'll pay about 50 cents an ounce for brands like Lucky Earth and Eco Touch. That comes to roughly $2 per wash.

The real truth about 'health' drinks

The market is flooded with enhanced waters and fortified drinks infused with extra vitamins, minerals, herbs, flavorings — and a hefty price tag. Are they worth it? Some specially formulated waters claim to rev up your energy, boost your immunity, or help you lose weight. See what's really in the bottles along with water.

Too few vitamins. You can buy water, juice, and soda with vitamins added, but often not enough to do a lot of good. Read the labels carefully to see how your favorite $2 bottle of water compares with the amount of vitamins in a glass of regular orange juice. Even worse, acid in the soft drinks causes the vitamins to break down. Not surprisingly, some of these beverages are loaded with sugar.

It's not clear how much good these vitamins do for you. Water-soluble vitamins, like vitamin C, may be more quickly absorbed from water than from solid food. But fat-soluble vitamins, like A, D, and E, enter your blood more easily if they're eaten with a little fat — not water.

Too much caffeine. Energy drinks, like Red Bull and Rockstar, make up the fastest-growing beverage group in the United States. They get most of their kick from sugar and caffeine. In fact, a 12-ounce serving of Red Bull contains 116 milligrams (mg) of caffeine — three times the caffeine in the same serving of cola. Then there are drinks that seem to have gone truly overboard, like Spike Shooter, with 428 mg of caffeine in 12 ounces. Some energy drinks also contain taurine, an amino acid that can help cut muscle fatigue after exercise. Unfortunately, energy drinks are reported to raise blood pressure and heart rate in some people.

Sports drinks, like Gatorade and Powerade, are among the worst beverages for your teeth. Their sugar and acid corrode tooth enamel more quickly than soda or fruit juice, although all three do damage. Your teeth will thank you for drinking water instead.

Too many calories. What could be better for weight loss than plain old water? Marketers want you to think products like Kellogg's

Special K2O Protein water or Airforce Nutrisoda Slender can help. But most are a mix of water, flavorings, vitamins, and artificial sweeteners. Some, like SoBe Life Water, actually contain almost as many calories as regular soda.

Instead of paying extra for a bottle of empty promises, many nutritionists suggest mixing an ounce of your favorite fruit juice into a glass of water for flavor and eating whole grains, low-fat dairy products, and fruits and vegetables to get all your nutrients.

Prevent a cold with 2 common items

Washing your hands with soap and water is the all-time best way to prevent a cold. You can fight 200 different viruses with these two items found in every kitchen and bathroom.

The common cold is caused by one of more than 200 different viruses, most commonly a form of rhinovirus or parainfluenza virus. These germs move from person to person when you shake hands, cough, sneeze, or touch an infected surface, like a stair railing. You can kill germs before they get a chance to make you sick by washing your hands often, especially during cold season. Here's the best way to get the job done.

- Use regular soap and running water for the most thorough cleaning.

- Rub your hands together to make a lather, scrubbing all surfaces. Do this for 20 seconds — enough time to sing "Happy Birthday" twice.

- Rinse your hands under warm, running water.

- Dry your hands with paper towels or an air dryer.

Whole grains

Head off high blood pressure

Switch from bland white rice to the nutty taste of brown rice, and you may never face the dangers of high blood pressure, heart attack, and stroke. Even better, you may miss out on the side effects of blood pressure drugs, too.

Focus on a grain-filled diet. It's no secret that diet can help after you get high blood pressure, but researchers from Boston's Brigham and Women's Hospital wanted to learn whether whole grains might help you avoid high blood pressure in the first place. To find out, they followed more than 28,000 women for 10 years. They discovered that women who ate at least four servings of whole grains were 23 percent less likely to get high blood pressure than women who ate little or none. These whole grains included foods like brown rice, popcorn, cooked oatmeal, dark breads, bran, and whole-grain breakfast cereals.

So what makes whole grains better than other grains? Consider the difference between white rice and brown rice. Like white bread and cake, white rice is a wimpy refined grain. That means the nutritious, fiber-filled outer layers of the grain have been stripped away, leaving the starchy part of the grain.

That's also why you usually need to flavor up white rice with butter, soy sauce, or other foods to hide its wishy-washy taste. But brown rice is different. It's a whole grain whose outer layers are never stripped away. That means you get the grain, the whole grain, and nothing but the grain — not to mention a lot more fiber, nutrients, and warm, hearty flavor.

> ### Super whole grains
>
> - ★ oats
> - ★ barley
> - ★ quinoa
> - ★ buckwheat
> - ★ bulgur
> - ★ millet
> - ★ whole wheat
> - ★ brown rice

Attack the causes of HBP. Scientists think the fiber in whole grains is the main reason these foods may prevent high blood pressure (HBP). In fact, fiber may attack several possible causes of high blood pressure, including obesity and insulin resistance.

■ Obesity may help promote high blood pressure by fouling up your body's ability to handle sodium or even by hampering the systems that regulate blood flow. But eating more fiber helps fill you up so you eat less. It may even help you absorb fewer calories from the fats and proteins you eat. As a result, you take in fewer calories and it's easier to lose weight.

---

7 simple fiber boosters

It doesn't take a whole lot of effort to get more whole grains into your diet. Just follow these simple tips.

- Enjoy a bowl of whole-grain cereal or oatmeal for breakfast.

- Make sandwiches with 100 percent whole-grain breads.

- Replace white rice with brown rice, barley, millet, buckwheat, bulgur, or quinoa.

- Bake with half white flour and half whole-wheat flour.

- Add 1/2 cup of cooked wheat or rye berries, wild rice, brown rice, or barley to soups.

- Mix 3/4 cup of uncooked oats with each pound of ground beef or turkey when making meatballs, burgers, or meatloaf.

- Snack on popcorn, or stir a handful of oats into your yogurt.

- Some studies suggest that insulin resistance helps your body retain more sodium. If that's true, that extra sodium may contribute to high blood pressure. But other studies have found that whole grains may lower insulin resistance by improving your body's ability to use insulin. That could not only protect you against high blood pressure, but diabetes, too.

So if you've been worried about high blood pressure, start adding more whole grains to your diet. Be sure to start slowly to give your body time to adjust without embarrassing side effects. With each extra serving of whole grains, you'll be cutting your danger of high blood pressure, heart attack, and stroke while raising the odds that you'll never need blood pressure drugs.

Battle belly fat and win

The #1 cause of big bellies is not beer or dessert. And it's probably on your table at least once every day. The good news is you may trim your waistline just by switching to a tastier alternative.

This diet downfall, believe it or not, is white bread. According to a study from Boston's Tufts University, people who eat more white bread increase their waist size three times faster than people who eat a healthy diet rich in whole grains. What's more, research from Pennsylvania State University found that dieters who ate more whole grains lost more body fat around the middle than dieters who ate refined grains. So making a simple change like switching from white bread to whole grain can help you trim your waist size.

If you combine eating more whole grains with eating less fat, you'll do even more to keep off the pounds that creep up over the years.

- People who cut fat and add fiber to their diets lose three times as much weight as those who merely cut the fat, according to a research review.

■ Many people gain weight as they age. But over eight years, men who ate more whole grains gained significantly less weight than men who scrimped on whole grains, a Harvard study says. And those men didn't even cut back on fats.

Eat this	Instead of this	For these benefits
fiber in whole grains, aim for 14 grams of fiber for every 1,000 calories you eat	simple carbohydrates, including refined grains and white bread	Fiber helps you feel full so you can avoid between-meal snacking and eat fewer calories to lose weight. Eating lots of fiber reduces your risk of developing diabetes. Soluble fiber may lower blood sugar. Adding whole grains to your diet may lower your blood pressure and cholesterol.
monounsaturated fats (MUFAs) such as olive oil	trans fats in shortening or some baked goods, saturated fats like butter and coconut oil	Trans fats encourage your body to pack on weight, especially around your belly. Meals with lots of saturated fats may cause a surge in triglycerides and cholesterol.
low-fat dairy	full-fat dairy	Get the protein and calcium you need without taking in too much saturated fat. Dairy products may encourage your body to lose weight, which may help ward off type 2 diabetes and heart disease.
fruit	sugar-filled snacks or desserts	Choose nutrient-dense foods rather than foods with lots of calories and few nutrients to avoid gaining weight.
water	soft drinks	Researchers found that people who trade regular soda for water tend to eat fewer calories in a day.
vegetables	red meat	Replace high-fat meat in your diet with fiber- and nutrient-filled vegetables to take in fewer calories and lose weight. Reduce your risk of colon cancer.

These simple secrets to eating right, shown in the table on the opposite page, can help control your weight more easily and protect your health. Just make these substitutions in your diet and you may dodge cancer, heart disease, diabetes, and weight problems. Anyone can do it.

3 ways grains fight heart disease

Centuries ago, the Leaning Tower of Pisa had perfectly even marble steps. But everyone who climbed the tower wore down the steps a little at a time. That wear took years to show, but today when you climb them you'll find deep dips in the stairs. A heart attack works the same way. At first, the wear and tear caused by our choices isn't noticeable, but later it may cause problems like high cholesterol, high blood pressure, heart attack, and stroke. Fortunately, whole grains can help resist that wear and tear in three ways.

Cuts cholesterol danger. According to a study published in the *American Journal of Clinical Nutrition,* people who eat the most whole grains have less LDL and total cholesterol than people who avoid whole grains. The fiber from oatmeal and other whole grains acts like a vacuum cleaner to suck cholesterol from your intestines and sweep it out of your body before you can absorb it into your bloodstream.

Controls your weight. The same study also found that whole-grain lovers have lower body mass indexes (BMI), smaller waists, and weigh less. This is good news because extra weight raises your risk of early death from heart disease, but trimming your waist measurement cuts your heart disease risk. What's more, reducing your BMI may lower your odds of high blood pressure.

Protects against artery trouble. Hardening of the arteries, or atherosclerosis, happens when plaque forms inside your artery walls, making those walls thicker and tougher. This can lead to narrowing of the arteries and high blood pressure — two potential causes of heart attack and stroke. According to a study from Wake Forest University, the more whole grains people ate, the less plaque they had in the common carotid artery — a major blood vessel in your neck. Scientists suspect some arteries may not benefit as much as others, so it's important to adopt as many heart-healthy habits as you can. But clearly, eating whole grains is a super place to start.

Best of all, you can get results from eating just a few servings of whole grains a day. Another study from Wake Forest University found that men who ate two or three servings of whole grains a day had 21 percent less risk of heart disease compared to people who rarely ate whole grains. Three servings isn't hard. Eat oatmeal for breakfast, a sandwich with whole-grain bread at lunch, and popcorn for a snack — and you'll have your three for the day.

Secret to defeating diabetes

Eating more, not less, could be the answer to improving your insulin sensitivity and heading off type 2 diabetes — as long as you're eating more whole grains.

In fact, you could lower your risk of type 2 between 20 and 30 percent just by packing at least two servings of whole grains into your day. And it's never too late to start. Experts say people who don't get enough now will benefit most from upping their intake.

In one study, overweight people with insulin problems were able to improve their insulin sensitivity after just six weeks of eating more whole grains. They didn't have to eat exotic foods, either. Most people ate whole wheat, rolled oats, and brown rice to fill their quota. Other research found whole grains lowered people's fasting and after-meal blood sugar. The secret lies in whole grains' combination of three special ingredients.

Magnesium. Magnesium plays a major role in how your body processes the sugar you get from foods. Experts also think this mineral helps balance your blood sugar and control the action of insulin in your body.

Bumping up your magnesium intake just 100 milligrams (mg) a day could cut your risk of type 2 diabetes 15 percent. That's the equivalent of four slices of whole-grain bread, one cup of beans, half a cup of cooked spinach, one-quarter cup of nuts, or four tablespoons of peanut butter. Simply swap whole-grain bread for white bread in sandwiches, or have a side of spinach with dinner instead of potato chips.

Aim for 325 mg of magnesium daily, a goal you can easily reach without supplements just by eating whole grains, beans, nuts, and leafy green vegetables. Getting more than 325 mg doesn't grant extra protection.

Fiber. In a review of nine studies, people who ate the most fiber — about 28 grams (g) a day — slashed their risk of type 2 diabetes by 14 percent compared to those who ate the least fiber, about 16 g a day. Scientists have two theories why.

- Soluble fiber slows the speed at which your stomach empties, so your bloodstream absorbs the sugar from food more slowly.

- Insoluble fiber doesn't completely digest in your stomach. Instead, it travels to your colon where it ferments, producing short-chain fatty acids. These compounds help make your cells more sensitive to insulin.

Chromium. This essential mineral may be essential to helping insulin work effectively, too. It is an ingredient in a substance called glucose tolerance factor and, as you might guess, a severe chromium deficiency leads to insulin resistance and diabetes. In theory, chromium could improve people's insulin sensitivity. People who don't have diabetes may not see a benefit from boosting their chromium levels, but it does seem to help those with type 2 by lowering fasting glucose levels and a substance called A1c, which shows blood-sugar average over time.

3-step plan thwarts type 2

Stop diabetes in its tracks with these three simple steps. There are no drugs and no starvation diets — no kidding. Just some common-sense advice on eating and living.

- Replace refined carbohydrates with high-fiber whole grains. People who eat mostly refined grains, like white rice or white bread, face a higher risk of diabetes, while eating whole grains can actually reduce your risk.

- Eat more healthy fats, like the monounsaturated kind in olive oil or the polyunsaturated fats in fish. Cut back on saturated fat in meat and trans fat in margarine and processed foods.

- Get moving. Exercise can help you shed extra pounds, whip your heart into shape, and avoid taking extra medications.

Easy way to keep cancer at bay

You can slash your risk of colon and intestinal cancers just by swapping white rice for brown, and refined grains for whole ones.

Researchers asked nearly 500,000 people ages 50 to 71 about their eating habits and health problems. High whole-grain eaters were 21 percent less likely to develop colon cancer.

- Humble whole grains like brown rice, oats, whole wheat, and barley are excellent sources of cancer-fighting nutrients, including minerals, B vitamins, vitamin E, and plant compounds called phenols.

- Whole-grain foods also help regulate blood sugar and insulin levels, which protects against colon and breast cancers.

- The insoluble fiber in grains may cut your risk of bowel cancers. It ferments in your gut, producing short-chain fatty acids which, in turn, squash the growth of tumors.

The keys here are whole grains. These cancer-busting nutrients generally reside in the outer bran layer. Refining whole grains into white rice or white flour, or white bread, strips most of these nutrients. For instance, processing removes up to 92 percent of the vitamin E in grain.

Thanks to its bran layer, brown rice may protect against intestinal cancer in a way white rice doesn't. Rice bran cut the incidence of cancerous intestinal tumors in half in a study on mice, leading researchers to think brown rice may help prevent cancer in people with intestinal polyps.

Give whole grains the green light in your diet, put refined grains on the back burner, and gain extra protection against digestive cancers.

Zinc

Zinc zaps colds and flu

Alphabetically, zinc comes last in the list of nutrients you need. But in terms of your health, this trace mineral ranks much higher. Zinc produces energy, makes DNA, helps your body use vitamin A, fights free radicals, heals wounds, and boosts your immune system.

That last function makes zinc a useful weapon against colds and flu. Boosting your zinc intake may boost your defenses against infection — especially if you're over age 55. A recent University of Michigan study found that seniors who took zinc supplements had fewer infections over one year. They also had lower levels of inflammation and oxidative stress, which takes its toll on your immune system. Even if they caught a cold, it only lasted about half as long — with less severe symptoms.

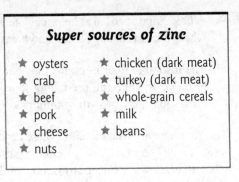

Super sources of zinc

- ★ oysters
- ★ crab
- ★ beef
- ★ pork
- ★ cheese
- ★ nuts
- ★ chicken (dark meat)
- ★ turkey (dark meat)
- ★ whole-grain cereals
- ★ milk
- ★ beans

Another study of nursing home residents found that those with low blood levels of zinc were more likely to get pneumonia. Those with normal levels fared much better. Researchers believe supplementing your diet to raise your zinc levels may help.

But don't rush out and buy a stockpile of zinc lozenges. While some studies show they help fight colds, most of the studies were poorly designed. Other studies have found no benefits for zinc lozenges. Using lozenges may not be worth the risk of side effects, including nausea, stomachache, and an unpleasant taste. Too much zinc can also lead to a malfunctioning of your immune system and chronic fatigue.

One well-designed study showed that zinc nasal gels may help reduce the duration and severity of colds, if you start using them within one or two days of the first sign of illness. Nevertheless, these products come with their own risks, including the possible loss of your sense of smell.

Age-proof your eyes

Zinc, a powerful antioxidant mineral, may fight age-related macular degeneration, the leading cause of vision loss in people over age 55 — but it may also contribute to it.

Macular degeneration affects the macula, the part of your retina that controls central vision, and gradually leads to blurred vision or a blind spot in the center of your visual field. You may have trouble picking out printed words and fine details, straight lines may appear wavy, and shapes may appear distorted.

Low levels of dietary zinc have been linked to an increased risk of developing age-related macular degeneration (AMD). In a Dutch study, those who had above-average consumption of zinc, beta carotene, and vitamins C and E had a 35 percent lower risk of AMD. Other studies show taking zinc supplements may help.

The Age-Related Eye Disease Study found that high doses of zinc, along with fellow antioxidants beta carotene, copper, and vitamins C and E, helped people with intermediate or advanced AMD. This treatment slowed the progression of AMD by 25 percent, but it did not prevent it.

Not all the news about zinc is good. A recent British study found that zinc may play a role in the development and progression of AMD. One sign of AMD is the build up of tiny deposits, called drusen, in the eye. The British researchers discovered surprisingly high levels of zinc in these deposits, indicating that too much zinc could be to blame.

Your safest bet for saving your vision is to get zinc through your diet, not by taking high doses of supplements. Don't take zinc supplements without talking to your doctor first.

Cushion your joints with key mineral

Nutrition plays an important role in maintaining healthy joints. Simply getting enough zinc into your diet may help protect you from arthritis.

Osteoarthritis, the most common form of arthritis, occurs when the cartilage that cushions your joints gradually wears away, and your bones rub together. With rheumatoid arthritis, your immune system goes haywire and attacks your joints, damaging your cartilage and bones.

People with osteoarthritis often have low zinc levels. Men should aim for 11 milligrams of zinc every day and women should strive for 8 mg — but vegetarians may need 50 percent more zinc than nonvegetarians. That's because your body has a harder time absorbing zinc from plant sources. However you get your zinc, this mineral also contributes to bone health, further boosting your defense against arthritis and even osteoporosis, or brittle bone disease.

Because of its anti-inflammatory properties, zinc may also fight rheumatoid arthritis. When paired with copper, zinc may be even more effective against this condition.

Wise up to zinc

You need zinc, but you can get too much of a good thing. High doses of supplemental zinc may lead to urinary problems in older people, according to a recent study. Researchers took a closer look at the Age-Related Eye Diseases Study in which 3,640 people ages 55 to 80 received either zinc, antioxidants, zinc plus antioxidants, or a placebo. Those taking zinc were more likely to be hospitalized for urinary complications, including urinary tract infections and urinary stones. Too much zinc can also lead to copper deficiency.

The recommended dietary allowance (RDA) for zinc is 8 milligrams (mg) for women and 11 mg for men. The tolerable upper intake level for zinc is 40 mg a day. People in the study received 80 mg a day.

Food secrets:
More nutrition
for less money

Slash your grocery bill

Americans waste about 27 percent of the food available to them. And it happens at all stages of the food chain, from growing, harvesting, preparing, and storing. Make the most of the food you buy with one of these new products created to help it last longer without spoiling.

- "Green bags." Several brands contain zeolite, a natural mineral that absorbs ethylene gas, which causes fruits and vegetables to ripen faster. Ten green bags cost about $5, and you can reuse them. Although test results vary, the bags seem to do a better job than regular plastic bags on certain foods, like bananas and strawberries.

- Vacuum-sealing systems. This method lets you wrap food tightly — with no air trapped inside to speed up spoilage. You can use it to package bulk meat into smaller portions, seal your garden-fresh veggies, or get more mileage out of leftovers. Systems start at around $50, and the vacuum sealing is supposed to make food last about five times longer.

- DaysAgo digital counter. This gadget keeps track of how long food has been in your refrigerator. Set the counter when you wrap up leftovers, and you'll know how long they've been hanging around.

Household Hint

Super way to soften sugar

Don't toss out that open bag of brown sugar, even if it's hardened into a rock-like lump. Place an apple slice in the bag overnight. That bit of moisture will soften up the brown sugar so it's soft, crumbly, and easy to use.

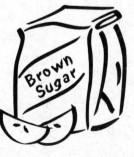

Lock in nutrients with careful cooking

Eating your vegetables raw is not always the healthiest choice. Depending on the food and the nutrients, certain cooking methods may actually make your food healthier. Some nutrients are frail, so high heat destroys them. Others sneak out into the cooking water. Still others remain tightly locked into the body of the produce until cooking releases them.

Carotenoids. Carrots, zucchini, and broccoli need a good boiling to make their carotenoids available. That's what researchers found when they compared boiling, stir-frying, and steaming. Longer cooking time softened these tough veggies, releasing the important nutrients.

Polyphenols. These colorful phytonutrients in red potatoes and purple cabbage wash out easily into the cooking water when boiled. Instead, eat these vegetables raw or stir-fry them quickly.

Vitamin C. This delicate water-soluble vitamin breaks down easily at high heat, so eat your bell peppers and broccoli raw to absorb this nutrient. One study found 87 percent of broccoli's vitamin C was lost in frying, while carrots lost 38 percent of their vitamin C during steaming and 100 percent in frying.

Lycopene. Many people eat tomatoes for their bright red carotenoid, lycopene. Tomatoes are actually a better source of this nutrient after they've been processed. As with the fat-soluble vitamins — vitamins A, D, E, and K — cooking breaks down the thick cell walls of plants to release the nutrients. Enjoy your tomatoes in sauce and ketchup.

Potassium. You can make potatoes cook faster if you shred or cube them before boiling, but doing so also lowers the amount of potassium you'll get from this tasty tuber.

Quercetin. Cook your onions in the microwave or a frying pan and they'll hold on to more quercetin, an important flavonoid. But boil onions and you're tossing 30 percent of their quercetin into the water.

Garlic. Raw garlic is a great source of allicin, but that phytonutrient gets lost when garlic is cooked whole. Crush the garlic before cooking and the allicin remains.

Spices. You can count on cinnamon, cloves, fennel, rosemary, and other herbs and spices to provide you with loads of antioxidants. Researchers found simmering and stewing gave these spices even more antioxidant power, while grilling and stir-frying reduced it.

Keep your food fresh longer

Rising food costs make it more painful to see those lovely berries turn into moldy sludge. Store each type of food properly to extend its shelf life.

Type of food	Best storage method	What you need to know
Fruit		
apples	refrigerate	cool temperatures won't harm flavor, which happens with other fruits
strawberries	hull, slice in half, freeze in sealed baggies	add sugar syrup to baggie to preserve bright red color of berries
bananas	buy green and let them ripen on counter	cold temperature of your refrigerator will cause them to turn black
oranges	store in refrigerator or at room temperature for same results	will last about two weeks either way, but they'll grow mold if stored in plastic
peaches	on counter in paper bag with a banana	ethylene gas from ripening banana encourages peaches to soften
Vegetables		
broccoli	refrigerate for up to seven days	loses only small amounts of glucosinolates, helpful compounds
corn	trim husks, remove silks and stalks; blanch for five minutes, then cool, dry, and freeze	buy fresh in season when price is low, save to eat during winter and spring, lasts for about a year

Type of food	Best storage method	What you need to know
Vegetables (continued)		
onions	store in a cool, dark place	keep separate from potatoes, since their moisture can make onions rot
spinach	buy it frozen if you plan to serve it cooked	fresh spinach loses nutrients quickly, while freezing locks them in
tomatoes	ripen at room temperature, eat within three days of ripening	refrigeration causes loss of flavor and texture
Dairy		
cheese	refrigerate to retain texture	buy it cheaper in bulk, then shred hard cheese and freeze for six to eight months
milk	refrigerate for up to a week after "sell by" date	buy it cheaper in bulk, pour off a glass, then seal and freeze; thaw in sink of water
yogurt	refrigerate for up to two weeks after "sell by" date	may separate when frozen
eggs	refrigerate for four to five weeks	fresh eggs last longer than pasteurized egg products and egg substitutes
Others		
uncooked whole oats, brown rice	freeze if you don't use within a week	exposure to air or heat may cause whole grains to become rancid
basil and other herbs	remove stems, then rinse, dry, and chop leaves; freeze in sealed baggie for six months	buy fresh in bulk when they're in season
vegetable oil	store in a cool, dark place	lasts one to three months after opening, so don't overbuy

10 most powerful foods on the produce aisle

Fill your grocery cart with these 10 powerhouse foods, and you have all the ingredients you need to protect your blood vessels, lower your cancer risk, keep your eyesight sharp, and more. They're bursting with fiber, vitamins, minerals, antioxidants, and natural plant chemicals to battle the most common health problems of aging.

Food	Health benefits	How it works
apples	aid digestion	soluble and insoluble fiber maintain digestive regularity
	prevent heart disease	flavonoids work as antioxidants to lower LDL cholesterol
avocados	prevent deep vein thrombosis	vitamin E acts as an anticoagulant to prevent clots
	battle high blood pressure	potassium balances sodium in diet to lower blood pressure
broccoli	prevents cancer	indoles and isothiocyanates activate enzymes that remove carcinogens
cherries	battle arthritis	anthocyanins reduce painful inflammation
garlic	lower high cholesterol	antioxidant effects of garlic lower LDL cholesterol
	fight high blood pressure	allicin acts as antioxidant to dilate blood vessels
grapes	keep away Alzheimer's disease	polyphenol antioxidants protect brain better than supplements
oranges	protect against arthritis	vitamin C encourages buildup of collagen, which is needed for healthy cartilage in joints
spinach	prevents stroke	folate lowers homocysteine levels, reducing stroke risk
	keeps away osteoporosis	manganese helps enzymes function to keep bones dense and strong

Food	Health benefits	How it works
sweet potatoes	keep your eyesight sharp	beta carotene, vitamin C, vitamin E, and zinc work as antioxidants to prevent age-related macular degeneration
	help avoid osteoporosis	potassium helps bones stay strong by holding on to calcium
tomatoes	lower cancer risk	lycopene and other nutrients work together to block cell damage

---

New frontiers for food safety

You hear news reports almost weekly of contaminated food making people sick. Here's what food safety experts are working on to minimize your risk.

- Edible food wraps. This spray-on wrap is made of fruit or vegetable puree with added herbal oil. It's supposed to help produce keep its flavor longer — and kill dangerous bacteria, including E. coli. Experts are still working to develop these products, which may add the flavors of the herbs used — like oregano or cinnamon — to fresh fruits and vegetables.

- Irradiation. The U.S. Food and Drug Administration (FDA) recently approved allowing food producers to use radiation to kill dangerous bacteria, like E. coli and Salmonella, that can contaminate fruits and vegetables. Some food experts worry irradiation may zap nutrients and taste, while creating dangerous chemicals, but the FDA says it's safe.

Index

A

Açai 1-3
Acetaminophen, and caffeine 89
Acetic acid 12
Acetylcholine, memory and 8
Acid reflux. *See* Heartburn
Acids, in citrus fruit 82
Acrylamides, reducing 247-248, 284
Adrenalin 46
Age-related macular degeneration (AMD)
  beta carotene for 39-40
  fish for 135
  goji berry for 157
  lutein and zeaxanthin for 187
  vitamin D for 320-321
  zinc and 350-351
Allergies, honey for 174-175
Almond milk 200
Alopecia 282
Alpha-linolenic acid. *See* Omega-3 fatty acids
Alzheimer's disease
  apples for 8
  coffee for 93-94
  curry powder for 112-113
  fish for 131-132
  grapes for 271-272
  high blood pressure and 57
  Mediterranean diet for 217
  vitamin A for 37
Alzheimer's gene 37
Anthocyanins
  in blood oranges 50
  in cherries 66
Anthrax 46
Anti-aging 74, 216-217, 329-330, 332

Antibiotics, green tea and 165
Ants, natural remedies for 80, 234, 314
Apple rings, drying 10
Apples 4-10, 358
Arrhythmia. *See* Irregular heartbeat
Arthritis
  açai for 2
  cabbage for 109
  capsaicin for 60
  cherries for 66
  ginger for 154-155
  osteo 183, 212, 268, 291, 307, 318, 351
  pomegranates for 241
  psoriatic 61
  rheumatoid 113, 135, 166, 352
  vitamin C for 86
Ascorbic acid. *See* vitamin C
Aspirin 11-17
  cranberries and 101
Asthma
  aspirin for 14
  fish for 138-139
  passion fruit for 230-231
  vitamin D for 323-324
Atherosclerosis 56
  garlic for 147
  olive oil for 212
  whole grains for 345
Autoimmune disorders, vitamin D for 321-322
Avocados 327, 358

B

Bacteria
  fiber and 54
  helpful 258

in lemons 86
in mouth 48, 100, 120, 161
in produce 19
in stomach 215
UTIs and 99
wine and 276
Bags, green, for food storage 354
Baking soda 17-22
Bananas 23-27
Bath
baking soda for 19
oatmeal for 209
Beans 28-33
Bee sting, baking soda for 18
Belly fat, and dementia 32
Benign prostatic hyperplasia
(BPH) 186, 223
Berry, goji 157-160
Beta amyloid 8, 94
Beta carotene 33-41
in cranberries 100
Beta glucan 203
Bicarbonate 22
Bing cherries 67
Bipolar disorder, fish oil for 134
Bird feeder 87
Birdseed, and peanut butter 87
Bites, natural remedies for 18-19,
208
Black tea 42-49
Bladder
cancer 104
infection 166
overactive 335
Blood clots, preventing 11, 74,
148, 211, 286
Blood orange 49-52
Blood pressure
magnesium for 191
potassium for 23
sodium and 23
vitamin D and 324

Blood sugar
balancing 95-97, 190, 206
inulin and 177
vinegar and 306
Blood thinners. *See also* Warfarin
goji berry and 159
turmeric and 113
Blueberries, omega-3 in 219
Body mass index (BMI) 53
Bone density, and chocolate 75
Bones. *See also* Osteoporosis
bananas for 26-27
building 226
calcium for 121-122
lycopene for 303-304
magnesium for 194
omega-3 for 219-220
onions for 225-226
soy for 294-296
tea for 42
vitamin D for 317-318
vitamin K for 109
Boron
for memory 9
for osteoarthritis 6
Botulism 41
Brain cancer, capsaicin for 63
Brain plaque 113
Brassicas. *See* Cruciferous
vegetables
BRAT diet 26
Breakfast cereal 52-59
Breakfast, and weight loss 53
Breast cancer
aspirin for 12-13
beans for 29
crucifers for 105-107
soy and 293-294
vitamin D for 316
Breathing problems. *See* Asthma;
Chronic obstructive pulmonary
disease (COPD)

Broccoli 358
  for immune system 110
Brown sugar, softening 354
Buffered aspirin, side effects of 16-17
Bug bites, natural remedies for 18-19, 208
Bug spray, homemade 65
Bulb syringe, for nasal irrigation 18
Burning mouth syndrome 62

C

Cabbage, for arthritis 109
Caffeine, acetaminophen and 89
Calcium
  for diabetes 118
  for gum disease 251
  for osteoporosis 121
  in eggshells 126
Cancer. *See also* specific cancers
  açai for 2
  aspirin for 13
  beans for 28-30
  capsaicin for 63
  charbroiled foods and 12-13
  cherries for 68
  citrus for 84-85
  cranberries for 102-103
  curry powder for 113-114
  garlic for 149, 222
  ginger for 155
  grapes for 272-273
  grilling and 269
  leafy greens for 183
  marinades and 307-308
  onions for 222
  plums for 235
  potatoes and 247-248
  sulforaphane for 106
  tea for 43
  vitamin A for 35-36
  vitamin C for 85
  vitamin D for 315-317

vitamin E and 330
  water for 336-337
  whole grains for 348-349
Canker sore, baking soda for 18
Capsaicin 59-66
Car wash, waterless 338
Carbohydrates 278
Carrots, varieties of 40
Cassia cinnamon 78
Cataracts
  curcumin for 115-116
  fish for 134-135
  lutein and zeaxanthin for 188
  vitamin C for 157, 228
Cauliflower, colored 108
Cavities
  cheese for 120
  probiotics for 256
  tea for 48, 160-161
Celiac disease 209
Cereal, breakfast 52-59
Ceylon cinnamon 78
Chaffed skin, cornstarch for 98
Charbroiled foods, and cancer
  risk 12-13
Cheese
  cavities and 120
  yak 119
Cherries 66-69, 358
Cherry pit pillow 69
Chestnuts 202
Chia seed. *See* Salba
Chicken salad 287
Chicken soup, for colds 150, 263-264
Chlorogenic acid, in coffee 89
Chocolate 69-76
Chocolate mousse 300
Cholesterol. *See also* High
  cholesterol
  in eggs 123-125
  soy and 292
Chromium, for diabetes 347

Chronic obstructive pulmonary
   disease (COPD) 9-10, 139
   beta carotene for 41
Chronic pain
   capsaicin for 59-60
   mouth and 62
   vitamin D and 317
Cider, apple 4
Cinnamon 77-80
Citrus 80-88
Cleaning
   coffee grounds for 95
   nontoxic 88
   with baking soda 21-22
   with beans 192
   with olive oil 216
   with onions and leeks 225
   with powdered milk 252
   with salt 333
   with tea 49, 163
   with vinegar 310-312
Cleanser, scented 22
Clogged drain 312
Cocoa
   cooking with 73
   for skin 74
   to fight disease 70
Cocoa powder 71
Coconut water 334
Coffee 88-95
Coffee grounds, for cleaning 95
Cola, and high blood pressure 93
Cold sores, vitamin C for 110
Colds
   chicken soup for 150, 263-264
   citrus for 80-81
   fish for 139-140
   garlic for 150
   prevention 340
   tea for 47
   vitamin E for 329
   zinc for 349-350

Collagen 229
Colloidal oatmeal 208
Colon cancer
   aspirin for 14
   beans for 29
   cherries for 68
   crucifers for 107-108
   curcumin for 114
   dairy for 122-123
   leafy greens for 186
   magnesium for 192-193
   olive oil for 214-215
   probiotics for 261-262
   selenium for 289-290
   vitamin D for 316
Colored cauliflower 108
Congestive heart failure, cereal for
   56
Constipation
   cereal for 57
   dried plums for 236
   fiber for 7
   honey for 169
   inulin for 176
   water for 332
Cornbread, flaxseed 146
Cornstarch 95-98
Cortisol 46
Cough, honey for 169
Coumarin 77
Cramps, muscle, magnesium for
   194
Cranberries 99-103
Cravings, food 229
Creams, topical 155
Crohn's disease 137, 263
Cruciferous vegetables 104-112
Curcumin
   for cancer 114
   for neuropathy 116
Curry powder 112-117

D

Daidzein 298
Dairy 117-123. *See also* Milk; Yogurt
Dandruff, aspirin for 13
Dark chocolate 71
DASH diet 192
Decaffeinated coffee 93
Decorating
  with beans 32
  with cranberries 103
  with produce 184
Deep vein thrombosis 129, 327
Deer repellent, natural 65
Dementia. *See also* Alzheimer's disease
  belly fat and 32
  cereal for 55
  fish for 132
  green tea for 164
Dental plaque 48, 81, 100
Dentin 81
Depression, fish for 133-134
Diabetes
  beans for 30-31
  calcium for 118
  capsaicin for 65-66
  cereal for 54
  chromium for 347
  citrus for 82-84
  coffee for 89-91
  cornstarch for 95-97
  curry powder for 114-116
  dairy for 117-118
  fiber for 347
  fish for 130-131
  garlic for 151
  grapes for 273
  green tea for 161-162
  inflammation and 65
  inulin for 177
  magnesium for 190-191
    Mediterranean diet for 217
    nuts for 201
    oatmeal for 206
    potatoes and 246-247
    probiotics for 256-257
    protein for 118
    selenium and 290
    sleep and 25
    vitamin D for 118, 325
    whole grains for 346-347
Diarrhea 8
    dietary fructose intolerance and 170
    fiber intake and 207
    irritable bowel syndrome and 25, 232
    magnesium and 193
Diet
    BRAT 26
    DASH 192
    low-salt 335-336
    Mediterranean 211, 216-217
Dietary fructose intolerance 170
Dieting. *See* Weight loss
Digestion, inulin for 176
DNA damage, carotenoids for 39
Docosahexaenoic acid (DHA) 128, 133
Drain, clogged 312
Dressing, salad 35
Dried plums 236-237
Drinks, energy 339
Driving fatigue, scents for 79
Dry skin, cornstarch for 98
Dyeing yarn 115
Dyspepsia. *See* Indigestion

E

E. coli 86, 151, 172, 235, 276. *See also* Food poisoning
Eggs 123-127
Eggshells, for plants 126

Eicosapentaenoic acid (EPA) 128, 133
Electrolytes 332-340
Energy drinks 339
Epsom salts 193
Exercise, and fish oil 136
Extra-virgin olive oil 213
Eyesight. *See* Vision

F

Fatigue, driving, scents for 79
Fats. *See* Monounsaturated fatty acids (MUFAs)
Feeder, bird 87
Fiber 245
  boosting 342
  daily goals 57
  for diabetes 82
  for irritable bowel syndrome 25, 207
  gut bacteria and 54
  in beans 28
  in cranberries 100
  insoluble 7, 53, 207
  mucilage 141
  soluble 7, 207, 347
  to lower cholesterol 5
Fireplace, cleaning 163
Fish 127-141
Fish oil
  exercise and 136
  supplements 138
Flaxseed 141-146
Floors, cleaning 49
Flu
  citrus for 80-81
  tea for 47
  zinc for 349-350
Fluoride 48
Folate
  for stroke 179

  in beans 30
  in citrus 85
  warning 181
Folic acid. *See* Folate
Food
  charbroiled 12
  cravings 229
  secrets 353-359
  storage 354, 356, 357
Food poisoning
  cranberries for 102
  fish and 130
  garlic for 150
  honey for 175
  mercury and 130
  oregano for 102
  preventing 359
  produce and 19
  rosemary for 284
Foods, top 10 358-359
Foot odor, baking soda for 21
Free radicals 28, 223
French paradox 270
Fructans 176
Fructose 171
Fructose malabsorption. *See* Dietary fructose intolerance
Fruit. *See also* Produce
  for weight loss 229
Fungi, cinnamon for 80

G

Gallstones, and turmeric 113
Garlic 147-152, 356, 358
Gastro-esophageal reflux disease (GERD), and peppermint 233
Genistein 292
Ginger 153-156
Gingivitis. *See* Gum disease
Glucose 161, 171. *See also* Blood sugar

Gluten 209
Glycemic Index (GI) 31, 83, 201, 246
Goji berry 157-160
Gout. *See also* Arthritis
    cherries for 66
Grains, whole 341-349
Grapes, red 270-276, 358
Green bags, for food storage 354
Green tea 160-168
Greens, leafy 179-187
Grilling, and cancer risk 12-13, 269, 308
Grocery bill, cutting 266, 354
Grooming, baking soda for 20-21
Grounds, coffee 95
Gum disease
    calcium for 251
    cranberries for 100
    heart disease and 252
    pomegranate for 242
    vitamin C for 81
    vitamin D for 319
Gum, cinnamon 77

H

H. pylori. See Helicobacter (H.) pylori
Hair
    flaxseed for 144
    herbs for 282
    olive oil for 214
    yogurt for 259
Hardening of the arteries. *See* Atherosclerosis
Hay fever, honey for 174-175
Hazelnuts 199
HDL cholesterol 219. *See also* High cholesterol
Headache. *See also* Migraine
    peppermint oil for 234
    water for 332
Health cereals, truth about 58

Hearing loss
    vitamin E for 331
    aspirin for 15
    magnesium for 194
    resveratrol for 273
Heart
    cranberries for 101
    curry powder for 117
    flaxseed for 141-143
    monounsaturated fatty acids for 211
    nuts for 198-200
    pomegranate for 239-240
    potatoes for 244-245
    quercetin for 221
    tomatoes for 301-302
    vinegar for 309-310
Heart disease
    açai for 1
    apples for 5
    beans for 31-32
    beta carotene for 34
    cereal for 56
    cherries for 67-68
    chocolate for 69-71
    coffee and 92-93
    eggs and 125
    fish for 127-129
    garlic for 148
    gum disease and 252
    honey for 173-174
    leafy greens for 179-180
    lutein for 189
    oatmeal for 203-205
    salba for 284-286
    soy for 292
    tea for 44
    vitamin C for 227
    vitamin D for 324
    vitamin E for 245, 326-327
    whole grains for 345-346
Heartbeat, irregular 128

Heartburn
  hot peppers for 61
  peppermint and 233
Helicobacter (H.) pylori
  cranberries for 99
  in stomach 215, 260
  probiotics and 259-261
Hemorrhagic stroke. *See also*
  Stroke
  fish and 129
Heparin, and turmeric 113
Herbs, for healing 280-282
Herperidin, in blood oranges 50
Heterocyclic amines (HCAs),
  reducing 12, 284, 308
High blood pressure
  Alzheimer's disease and 57
  bananas for 23-24
  cereal for 57
  cinnamon for 79
  coffee and 93
  cola and 93
  cranberries for 101
  dark chocolate for 71-72
  flaxseed for 142
  garlic for 147
  grapes for 270
  melatonin for 23-24
  oatmeal for 204
  olive oil for 211
  omega-3 for 128, 217-218
  passion fruit for 227
  potassium for 245
  salba for 285
  salt and 336
  tea for 45
  tomatoes for 301
  whole grains for 341-343
High blood sugar.
  See Hyperglycemia
High cholesterol
  apples for 5

beans for 32
beta carotene for 33
cinnamon for 79
cranberries for 101
flaxseed for 141-142
garlic for 147
grapes for 271
oatmeal for 203
olive oil for 211
omega-3 for 218-219
tea for 44
vitamin D for 324
whole grains for 345
Hip fractures 42
Hives, cornstarch for 98
Honey 169-175
Hormone replacement therapy,
  substitute for 143
Hormone-free meat 268
Hot flashes
  flaxseed for 143
  soy for 298
Hot peppers, and capsaicin 59-60
Hot sauce, for pests 65
Hyperglycemia 96
Hypertension. *See* High blood
  pressure
Hypoallergenic egg 125
Hypoglycemia, cornstarch for 96

I

IBS. *See* Irritable bowel syndrome
  (IBS)
Immune system
  broccoli for 110-111
  fish for 139-140
  garlic for 150
  probiotics for 253-254
  tea for 47
  vitamin C for 228-229
  vitamin E for 327-329

Impotence, pomegranate for 243
Indigestion
    hot peppers for 61
    peppermint for 232
Indole-3-carbinol 106
Indonesian cinnamon 78
Infection
    cranberries for 99
    garlic for 150
    honey for 171-172
    tea for 47, 166
    zinc for 349-350
Inflammation
    cherries for 66
    curry powder for 113
    depression and 134
    diabetes and 65
    flaxseed for 142
    ginger for 154-155
    grapes for 271
    green tea for 166
    gums and 81
    olive oil for 212
    onions for 221-222
    Parkinson's disease and 14-15
    vitamin D for 320
Inflammatory bowel disease
    (IBD). See Crohn's disease;
    Ulcerative colitis
Influenza. See Flu
Insoluble fiber
    for diabetes 347
    in cereal 53
    irritable bowel syndrome and 207
Insomnia
    cherries for 67
    honey for 171
Insulin 118
Insulin resistance 31, 90
Interleukin-6 38
Intrinsic factor 133
Inulin 176-178

Irregular heartbeat 128
Irrigation, nasal 17-18
Irritable bowel syndrome (IBS)
    bananas for 25-26
    fiber for 207
    peppermint oil for 232
    potatoes for 248-249
    probiotics for 258
Ischemic stroke. See also Stroke
    aspirin and 11
    fish for 129
Isoflavones 294, 297
Isothiocyanates (ITCs)
    for breast cancer 106
    in cruciferous vegetables 104
Itchy skin, soothing 98, 208

J

Jet lag, melatonin for 67
Joints, painful. See Osteoarthritis
Juice
    carrot, storing 41
    cranberry, for UTIs 99
    grape, for dyeing 275
    lemon, for fish odor 141
    mangosteen, buying 196
    orange, for bones 87
    pomegranate, and weight 240

K

Kale 179
Kidney problems
    aspirin and 15
    magnesium and 193
Kidney stones
    turmeric and 113
    vitamin C and 84
    water and 332
Knee surgery, aspirin for 16

L

Laundry, baking soda for 20
LDL cholesterol 204, 239. *See also*
  High cholesterol
Leafy greens 179-187
Leeks
  for cleaning 225
  for prostate 224
Legumes. *See* Beans
Lemon
  bacteria and 86
  for cleaning 88
  for fish odor 141
  tea and 43, 167
Lignans 142
Limonoids, in citrus 85
Linoleic acid. *See* Omega-6 fatty
  acids
Liver cancer, and coffee 89
Low blood sugar. *See*
  Hypoglycemia
Low-salt diet 335-336
Lung cancer
  capsaicin for 63
  soy for 296
  vitamin D for 316
Lutein
  for heart 189
  for vision 187-189
Lycopene 228, 303, 355

M

Macadamias 198
Macular degeneration. *See* Age-
  related macular degeneration
Magnesium 190-195
  for diabetes 346-347
  in cereal 58
Mangosteen 195-198
Manuka honey 171-173
Marinade 222, 308

Meat tenderizer, for bee sting 19
Meat, hormone-free 268
MediHoney 171-173
Mediterranean Diet 211, 216-217
Melanoma. *See* Skin cancer
Melatonin
  for high blood pressure 23-24
  for irritable bowel syndrome 25
  for sleep 24
  in cherries 67
Memory
  acetylcholine and 8
  apples for 8
  chocolate for 72
  curry powder for 113
  fish for 131-133
  grapes for 271
  green tea for 164
  leafy greens for 180
  peppermint for 232
  pomegranates for 241
  rosemary for 279
Memory loss. *See also* Alzheimer's
  disease; Dementia
  soy and 299
Menopause
  flaxseed for 143
  soy for 298
Mercury poisoning 130
Metabolic syndrome 6
Migraine
  flaxseed for 144
  magnesium for 194
Milk
  almond 200
  powdered 249-253
  tea and 43
Milk chocolate 71
Milk of Magnesia 192
Mitochondria 63
Monounsaturated fatty acids
  (MUFAs), for heart 211
Motion sickness, ginger for 153

Mouth, bacteria in 48, 161
Mouthwash
    baking soda 18, 21
    honey 172
    mangosteen 197
Mucilage 141
Multiple sclerosis, fish for 140
Muscle
    cramps, magnesium for 194
    spasms 232
    strength, nutrients for 38, 288-
        289, 318
    weakness. *See* Sarcopenia

N

Naringenin, in blood oranges 50
Nasal irrigation 17-18
Nausea, ginger for 153
Nerve pain, capsaicin for 60
Neti pot, for nasal irrigation 18
Neuralgia. *See* Nerve pain
Neuropathy
    curcumin for 116
    resveratrol for 274
Nontoxic cleaning 88
Nose rinse. *See* Nasal irrigation
Nutrients, and cooking 355
Nuts 198-203

O

Oatmeal 203-210
Obesity. *See* Weight loss
Oil, flaxseed, storing 145
Olive oil 211-217
Omega-3 fatty acids 217-221. *See
    also* Fish; Flaxseed
Omega-6 fatty acids 220
    depression and 134
Onions 221-226, 355
Oral bacteria 48, 100, 120, 161
Orange 358

blood 49-52
juice, for bones 87
Oregano, for food poisoning 102
Osteoarthritis (OA). *See also*
    Arthritis
    boron for 6
    olive oil for 212
    protein for 268-269
    selenium for 291
    vinegar for 307
    vitamin D for 318-319
    vitamin K for 183
    zinc for 351-352
Osteoporosis
    bananas for 26-27
    chocolate and 75
    cinnamon for 79
    dairy for 121-122
    magnesium for 194
    omega-3 for 219-220
    plums for 236-237
    tea for 42
    vitamin C for 86-87
    vitamin D for 317-318
Ovarian cancer
    coffee for 89
    cranberries for 103
    tea for 44
    vitamin D for 316
Oven, cleaning 22
Overactive bladder 335
Oxalates 75
Oxygen radical absorbance capacity
    (ORAC) 1, 235

P

Pain, chronic. *See* Chronic pain
Pancreatic cancer
    curcumin for 114
    onions for 222-223
    vitamin D for 316
Parkinson's disease, aspirin for 14

Passion fruit 226-231
Peanut butter
 bars 238
 birdseed and 87
Peanuts 199
Pectin
 for cancer 4
 to lower cholesterol 5
Peppermint 232-234
 for driving 79-80
Periodontitis 81
Peripheral arterial disease 327
Personal care
 baking soda for 20-21
 oatmeal for 208-209
 olive oil for 214
Pests
 garlic for 152
 hot sauce for 65
Pillow, cherry pit 69
Pistachios 198
Plants, eggshells for 126
Plaque
 dental 48, 81, 100
 in arteries 44, 56, 190
 in brain 57, 113, 164
Plumegranate 242
Plums 235-238
Poison ivy, cornstarch for 98
Polychlorinated biphenyls (PCBs)
 130
Pomace oil 213
Pomegranate 239-244
Potassium
 for blood pressure 23
 in cranberries 100
Potatoes 244-249, 283
Powdered milk 249-253
Proanthocyanidins (PACs) 99, 103
Probiotics 253-263
Produce
 antioxidant levels 26
 food poisoning and 19

local 182
 washing 19
Prostate
 leafy greens for 186
 onions and leeks for 223-224
Prostate cancer
 crucifers for 111-112
 curcumin for 114
 dried tomatoes for 304-305
 fish for 140
 flaxseed for 143-144
 legumes for 29
 tea for 166-167
 vitamin D for 317
Protein 263-269
 for diabetes 118
Prunes. See Dried plums
Psoriasis
 capsaicin for 61
 omega-3 for 220
Psoriatic arthritis 61
Pudding, rice 76

Q

Quercetin
 for asthma 9
 for cancer 4
 for heart 221
 in cranberries 102

R

Recipes
 blood orange salad 52
 chicken salad 287
 chocolate mousse 300
 chocolate rice pudding 76
 cornbread 146
 curry fries 116
 fruit smoothie 253
 ginger salsa 156
 goji oatmeal crunch 160

Recipes *(continued)*
   green tea cheese dip 168
   ingredient substitutes 97
   oatmeal cookies 210
   peach apple crisp 3
   peanut butter bars 238
   pomegranate viniagrette 244
   rice cereal 59
   roasted potatoes 283
   vinegar dressing 309
Red grapes 270-276, 358
Repellent, deer 65
Resistant starch 248, 276-279
Restless legs syndrome (RLS),
   magnesium for 194
Resveratrol 270
Retinopathy 115
Rheumatoid arthritis (RA). *See also*
   Arthritis
   curry powder for 113
   fish for 135-136
   tea for 166
   zinc for 352
Rice pudding 76
Rinse, nose. *See* Nasal irrigation
Rosacea 208
Rosemary 279-284

S

Salad
   apricot and blood orange 52
   chicken 287
   dressing 35
   healthy choices 185
Salba 284-287
Salicylic acid. *See* Aspirin
Salt, cleaning with 333
Sarcopenia 38, 264-266, 288
Scented cleanser 22
Scurvy 81
Selenium 288-291
Shellfish, minerals in 133

Shingles, capsaicin for 60
Shoes, polishing 27
Shortening, substitution for 30
Silverfish 80
Sinusitis, nasal irrigation for 17-18
Skin
   açai for 2
   baking soda for 19, 21
   capsaicin for 61
   cornstarch for 97-98
   honey for 173
   itchy 98, 208
   mangosteen for 198
   oatmeal for 208
   olive oil for 214
   tomatoes for 302-303
   vitamin C for 229
   yogurt for 259
Skin cancer
   capsaicin for 63
   curcumin for 114
   green tea for 162-163
Sleep problems. *See also* Insomnia
   bananas for 24
   diabetes and 25
Smoking, and beta carotene 41
Smoothie, fruit 253
Snack bars, with resistant starch 277
Sneakers, freshening 98
Sodium, and blood pressure 23
Soluble fiber
   for diabetes 347
   for irritable bowel syndrome 207
Soy 292-300
Spastic colon. *See* Irritable bowel
   syndrome (IBS)
Spinach 358
Sports drinks 339
Stains, baking soda for 20
Starch, resistant 248, 276-279
Stings, baking soda for 18-19
Stomach, *H. pylori* and 215, 260
Storage, food 354, 356, 357

Stress
    tea for 45-46
    vitamin C for 83
Stroke
    aspirin for 11
    carotenoids for 34
    fish for 129
    folate for 179
    hemorrhagic 129
    ischemic 11, 129
    vitamin C for 227
Substance P 60, 61
Sugar, brown, softening 354
Sulforaphane
    for cancer 106
    for immune system 111
    sunscreen and 105
Sun damage 74, 242-243. *See also*
    Wrinkles
Sunburn, cornstarch for 98
Sunscreen, and sulforaphane 105
Sunshine, vitamin D from 315, 325
Surgery, knee, aspirin for 16
Sweet potatoes 359

T

Tabasco sauce, for burning mouth
    syndrome 62
Tea
    black, benefits of 42-49
    ginger 154
    green, benefits of 160-168
    milk and 43
    peppermint 232
Tea leaves, for ashes 163
Teeth, and citrus fruit 82
Tomatoes 301-305, 359
Toothpaste
    baking soda 21
    cinnamon 77
    for fish odor 141
Top 10 foods 358-359

Topical creams 155
Torrefacto-roasted coffee 91
Trans fats 344
Triglycerides 219
    omega-3 for 128, 131
True cinnamon 78
Turmeric
    dyeing with 115
    warnings about 113
Types of cinnamon 78

U

Ulcerative colitis 137, 263
    inulin for 176
Ulcers
    aspirin and 15
    capsaicin for 62
    cranberries for 99
    H. pylori and 259-260
Ultraviolet (UV) rays 74
Upset stomach. *See* Indigestion
Urinary problems, and zinc 352
Urinary tract infection (UTI)
    cranberry juice for 99
    garlic for 151
Ursolic acid, in cranberries 102
Uterine prolapse 57

V

Vacuum-sealing, for food storage
    354
Varicose veins, vitamin K for 183
Vegetables. *See also* Produce
    cruciferous 104-112
Vinegar 306-314
    for deodorizing 22
    from aspirin 12
Vision
    beta carotene for 39-40
    fish for 134-135
    goji berry for 157

Vision *(continued)*
   lutein and zeaxanthin for 187-189
   pomegranates for 241
   vitamin D for 320-321
Vitamin A
   for Alzheimer's disease 37
   for cancer 35-36
   supplement risk 36
Vitamin B12
   for stroke 129
   in seafood 132
Vitamin C
   for arthritis 86
   for bones 109
   for cancer 85
   for cataracts 228
   for cold sores 110
   for diabetes 83-84
   for heart disease 227
   for immune system 228-229
   for osteoporosis 86-87
   for skin 229
   for stroke 227
   for teeth and gums 81
   in blood oranges 51
   in cranberries 100
   kidney stones and 84
Vitamin D 315-325
   for diabetes 118
   for osteoporosis 122
Vitamin E 326-331
   in cranberries 100
Vitamin K
   for osteoarthritis 183
   for varicose veins 183
   in cabbage 109-110
   in kale 179

W

Walnuts 199
Warfarin
   garlic and 148
   ginger and 155
   turmeric and 113
Water 332-340
Waterless car wash 338
Weight loss
   beans for 31
   caffeine for 90
   capsaicin for 64
   cereal and 52-53
   eggs for 126-127
   fish oil for 136
   fruit for 229
   inulin for 178
   Mediterranean diet for 217
   nuts for 202
   oatmeal for 205
   protein for 267
   resistant starch and 278
   soy for 293
   vitamin D and 323
   water for 334-335
   whole grains for 343-345
   yogurt for 119-120
White chocolate 71
Whole grains 341-349
Wolfberry. *See* Goji berry
Wrinkles 208

Y

Yak cheese 119
Yam fries with curry 116
Yarn, dyeing 115
Yogurt
   for weight loss 119-120
   inulin in 178
   probiotics in 254

Z

Zeaxanthin, for vision 187-189
Zinc 349-352